P9-ARZ-787

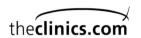
theclinics.com

PSYCHIATRIC CLINICS
OF NORTH AMERICA

Administrative Psychiatry: Advancing Quality Care

GUEST EDITORS
Daniel R. Wilson, MD, PhD
Peter F. Buckley, MD

March 2008 • Volume 31 • Number 1

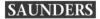
SAUNDERS
An Imprint of Elsevier, Inc.
PHILADELPHIA   LONDON   TORONTO   MONTREAL   SYDNEY   TOKYO

W.B. SAUNDERS COMPANY
A Division of Elsevier Inc.

1600 John F. Kennedy Boulevard • Suite 1800 • Philadelphia, PA 19103-2899

http://www.theclinics.com

PSYCHIATRIC CLINICS OF NORTH AMERICA   Volume 31, Number 1
March 2008   ISSN 0193-953X
Editor: Sarah E. Barth   ISBN-13: 978-1-4160-5869-4
     ISBN-10: 1-4160-5869-9

The ideas and opinions expressed in *Psychiatric Clinics of North America* do not necessarily reflect those of the Publisher. The Publisher does not assume any responsibility for any injury and/or damage to persons or property arising out of or related to any use of the material contained in this periodical. The reader is advised to check the appropriate medical literature and the product information currently provided by the manufacturer of each drug to be administered, to verify the dosage, the method and duration of administration, or contraindications. It is the responsibility of the treating physician or other health care professional, relying on independent experience and knowledge of the patient, to determine drug dosages and the best treatment for the patient. Mention of any product in this issue should not be construed as endorsement by the contributors, editors, or the Publisher of the product or manufacturers' claims.

Psychiatric Clinics of North America (ISSN 0193-953X) is published quarterly by Elsevier Inc., 360 Park Avenue South, New York, NY 10010-1710. Months of issue are March, June, September, and December. Business and Editorial Offices: 1600 John F. Kennedy Blvd., Suite 1800, Philadelphia, PA 19103-2899. Customer Service Office: 6277 Sea Harbor Drive, Orlando, FL 32887-4800 Periodicals postage paid at New York, NY and additional mailing offices. Subscription prices are $213.00 per year (US individuals), $362.00 per year (US institutions), $107.00 per year (US students/residents), $255.00 per year (Canadian individuals), $440.00 per year (Canadian Institutions), $297.00 per year (foreign individuals), $440.00 per year (foreign institutions), and $149.00 per year (international & Canadian students/residents). Foreign air speed delivery is included in all *Clinics*' subscription prices. All prices are subject to change without notice. **POSTMASTER:** Send address changes to *Psychiatric Clinics of North America*, Elsevier Periodicals Customer Service, 6277 Sea Harbor Drive, Orlando, FL 32887-4800. Customer Service: 1-800-654-2452 (US). From outside of the US, call 1-407-563-6020. Fax: 1-407-363-9661. E-mail: Journals CustomerService-usa@elsevier.com.

Psychiatric Clinics of North America is covered in *Index Medicus, Current Contents/Social and Behavioral Sciences, Social Science Citation Index, Embase/Excerpta Medica,* and PsycINFO.

Printed in the United States of America.

ELSEVIER
SAUNDERS

PSYCHIATRIC CLINICS
OF NORTH AMERICA

Administrative Psychiatry: Advancing Quality Care

GUEST EDITORS

DANIEL R. WILSON, MD, PhD, Professor and Chairman of Psychiatry, Professor of Anthropology, Creighton University Medical Center, Omaha, Nebraska

PETER F. BUCKLEY, MD, Professor and Chairman, Department of Psychiatry and Health Behavior, Medical College of Georgia, Augusta, Georgia

CONTRIBUTORS

BYRON BAIR, MD, Professor of Geriatric Internal Medicine, Professor of Geriatric Psychiatry, and Associate Director, Geriatric Research Education and Clinical Center, University of Utah School of Medicine, Salt Lake City Veterans Administration Hospital, Salt Lake City, Utah

ERIK BARROWS, MS, Enterprise Computing, University of Connecticut Health Center, Farmington, Connecticut

SUBHASH C. BHATIA, MD, Chief, Mental Health and Behavioral Sciences Department, VA Nebraska-Western Iowa Health Care System; and Professor and Vice-Chair for Clinical Affairs, Department of Psychiatry, Creighton University, Omaha, Nebraska

JAMES A. BOURGEOIS, OD, MD, Alan Stoudemire Professor of Psychiatry & Behavioral Sciences, Director, Psychosomatic Medicine Service, University of California, Davis, Sacramento, California

PETER F. BUCKLEY, MD, Professor and Chairman, Department of Psychiatry and Health Behavior, Medical College of Georgia, Augusta, Georgia

HATTIE C. COBB, BA, Postgraduate Researcher, Department of Psychiatry Behavioral Sciences, University of California, Davis, Sacramento, California

MICHAEL T. COMPTON, MD, MPH, Assistant Professor, Department of Psychiatry and Behavioral Sciences; and Department of Family and Preventive Medicine, Emory University School of Medicine, Atlanta, Georgia

PRAVEEN P. FERNANDES, MD, Assistant Professor, Department of Psychiatry, Creighton University; and Medical Director Ambulatory Psychiatry, Omaha, VA Medical Center, Omaha, Nebraska

DONALD M. HILTY, MD, Associate Professor and Vice-Chair of Faculty Development, Department of Psychiatry & Behavioral Sciences, University of California, Davis, Sacramento, California

MICHAEL F. HOGAN, PhD, Commissioner, New York State Office of Mental Health, Albany, New York; and Adjunct Professor, Case Western Reserve University, Cleveland, Ohio

JEANIE KNOX HOUTSINGER, BA, Academic Affairs Coordinator, Department of Psychiatry, Western Psychiatric Institute and Clinic; and Deputy Director, Robert Wood Johnson Foundation National Program Depression in Primary Care: Linking Clinical and System Strategies, University of Pittsburgh School of Medicine, Pittsburgh, Pennsylvania

ROGER G. KATHOL, MD, Adjunct Professor, Internal Medicine and Psychiatry, University of Minnesota Medical School, Minneapolis; and President, Cartesian Solutions, Inc., Burnsville, Minnesota

DONNA J. KEYSER, PhD, MBA, Management Scientist, RAND Corporation; and Associate Director, RAND-University of Pittsburgh Health Institute, Pittsburgh, Pennsylvania

TED LAWLOR, MD, Assistant Professor of Psychiatry; and Clinical Chief and Vice Chairman, Department of Psychiatry, University of Connecticut Health Center, Farmington, Connecticut

VISHAL MADAAN, MD, MBBS, Resident Instructor in Psychiatry, Department of Psychiatry and Child Psychiatry, Creighton University/University of Nebraska Medical Center, Omaha, Nebraska

STEVE MELEK, BA, Principle, Actuary, Milliman, Inc., Denver, Colorado

STUART MUNRO, MD, Associate Professor and Chair of Psychiatry, University of Missouri-Kansas City School of Medicine, Kansas City, Missouri

JONATHAN D. NEUFELD, PhD, Assistant Clinical Professor of Psychiatry & Behavioral Sciences, University of California, Davis, Sacramento, California

HAROLD ALAN PINCUS, MD, Senior Scientist, RAND Corporation; Director, Robert Wood Johnson Foundation National Program Depression in Primary Care: Linking Clinical and System Strategies, University of Pittsburgh School of Medicine, Pittsburgh, Pennsylvania; and Vice Chair for Strategic Initiatives and Director of Quality and Outcomes Research, Department of Psychiatry, Columbia University, New York-Presbyterian Hospital, New York, New York

SUSAN SARGENT, MBA, Vice President and Advisory Senior, Array Healthcare Facilities Solutions, King of Prussia, Pennsylvania

STEPHEN C. SCHEIBER, MD, Adjunct Professor, Department of Psychiatry and Behavioral Sciences, Northwestern University Feinberg School of Medicine, Chicago, Illinois

GEORGE E. TESAR, MD, Chairman, Department of Psychiatry & Psychology, Cleveland Clinic Neurological Institute, Cleveland Clinic Foundation, Cleveland, Ohio

KATHERINE WATKINS, MD, MSHS, Senior Natural Scientist, RAND Corporation, Santa Monica, California

DANIEL R. WILSON, MD, PhD, Professor and Chairman of Psychiatry, Professor of Anthropology, Creighton University Medical Center, Omaha, Nebraska

PETER M. YELLOWLEES, MD, MRCP, Professor of Clinical Psychiatry & Behavioral Sciences, Director of Academic Information Systems, University of California, Davis, Sacramento, California

PSYCHIATRIC CLINICS
OF NORTH AMERICA

Administrative Psychiatry: Advancing Quality Care

CONTENTS VOLUME 31 • NUMBER 1 • MARCH 2008

> A remarkable new analysis of mental health policy provides a lucid perspective on the status and impact of changes in mental health. The monograph is a systematic attempt to answer two questions: are people with a mental illness better off today than a generation ago, and if so why? This article considers that analysis and the prospects for transforming mental health care.

> After sharing several case examples of health care for patients who have mental health/substance use disorders (MH/SUDs) in the current health care environment, this article describes the advantages that would occur if assessment and treatment of MH/SUDs became a clinical, administrative, and financial part of physical health with common provider networks, the ability to combine service locations (integrated clinics and inpatient units), similar coding and billing procedures, and a single funding pool. Because transition to such a system is complicated, the article then describes several process changes that would be required for integrated service delivery to take place.

> If psychiatrists are to bring value to the health care team, training a renewable force of such psychiatrists is essential. Have psychiatrists been trained to bring maximal value to the health care team? Is such training being provided now? Given the current health care climate, will sufficient funding be available to train this renewable force optimally? This article addresses these questions from an historical-developmental perspective, identifies current challenges, and outlines opportunities for further growth and development.

This article describes the two major phenomena that shaped the overall findings of the Institute of Medicine report *Improving the Quality of Health Care for Mental and Substance Use Conditions* and that informed its overarching recommendations. These phenomena are (1) the co-occurrence of mental health, substance use, and general health conditions; and (2) differences in the delivery of services for mental health/substance use and general health care. It describes efforts currently underway that address these differences and might significantly improve delivery and outcomes of mental health/substance use services.

During the last decade, the Department of Veterans Affairs (VA) has made major strides in enhancing quality of medical, surgical, and mental health care for veterans. These improvements have been achieved through the will and commitment of VA leadership and by changes in the administrative structure, such as through the creation of Veteran Integrated Service Networks and patient care service lines, the use of state-of-the-art technology for electronic health records, implementation of high-value preventative and chronic disease management performance measures, and the ability to track their effectiveness. Parallel with these changes, the quality of mental heath care in the VA has also improved, as have mental health education and research.

This overview describes the application of primary, secondary, and tertiary prevention—as well as universal, selective, and indicated preventive interventions—to psychiatric and substance use disorders. Ways in which the psychiatrist with a clearly defined administrative role, such as the medical director of a program, service, agency, or organization, or a psychiatrist in some other directorial role (eg, director of education or clinical program director), can apply the prevention paradigm are described. Specifically, a prevention orientation is relevant to administrative psychiatry in the domains of service delivery, education and training, research, and community consultation and advocacy.

Telepsychiatry Reduces Geographic Physician Disparity in Rural Settings, But Is It Financially Feasible Because of Reimbursement?

Donald M. Hilty, Hattie C. Cobb, Jonathan D. Neufeld, James A. Bourgeois, and Peter M. Yellowlees

Telemedicine has been shown to improve rural patient outcomes in two randomized controlled trials, to increase access to many patients, to serve underserved minorities, and to train primary care providers. Yet, programs are dwindling even after successful grants due to inadequate reimbursement. Studies have been thoroughly done to gauge the payor status of potential rural telemedicine patients, as the "floodgates" are not generally open to all—including those who cannot pay—in typical grants. Or the population of one community may not be representative of others. This study is part of a grant that explored the use of telemedicine for rural service delivery, attempted to get a clear snapshot of whom would be served if all were invited (paying or not), and to understand issues with the reimbursement systems. This article (1) examines the receipts of reimbursement and insurance coverage during the 1-year grant period by determining actual versus projected reimbursements, (2) identifies what payor(s) typical patients use, and (3) identifies problems and barriers for future study. Other administrative issues pertinent to telemedicine and costs are briefly discussed (eg, no-show rates, staffing, scheduling).

Behavioral Health Electronic Medical Record

Ted Lawlor and Erik Barrows

The electronic medical record (EMR) will be an important part of the future of medical practice. Behavioral health treatment demands certain additions to the capabilities of a standard general medical EMR. The current focus on the quality management and financial aspects of the EMR are only initial examples of what this tool can do. It is important for behavioral health practitioners to understand that they must embrace this innovation and mold it into a product that serves their needs and the needs of their patients. An efficient and effective EMR will greatly assist the overall clinical enterprise in a number of important areas.

Leadership and Professional Workforce Development

Peter F. Buckley and Vishal Madaan

On an average, 4% of medical students from medical schools in the United States choose psychiatry as an option. Although in recent years psychiatry residency match statistics have improved, in general terms it is less competitive to enter this specialty. Most psychiatrists practice as generalists, either in private practice or in the public mental health system. There are marked shortages in child psychiatry and in upcoming new subspecialties. There are ongoing efforts to enhance the core competency of psychiatrists-in-training, with particular emphasis on research literacy to foster lifelong learning skills and (for some) to stimulate interest in a research career track. This article chronicles the trajectory of workforce development and professional growth in psychiatry.

The American Board of Psychiatry and Neurology (ABPN) is a non-profit organization founded in 1934 to serve the public interest and promote excellence in the practice of psychiatry and neurology. The ABPN is one of 24 American Board of Medical Specialties boards that have helped develop processes that identify qualified specialists through rigorous credential and training requirements and successful completion of respective certification examinations. The ABPN has had an enormous influence on the practice of psychiatry in America and the world and this influence continues to grow. Here we provide an historical overview of the ABPN, its formation, mission, roles, and changes that have taken place over the years in the certification, recertification, and maintenance of certification process.

Psychiatrists have formed organizations for more than 100 years. The focuses of these organizations include education, clinical specialty, research, treatment modality, and psychiatrist identity. Psychiatrists in Canada and Britain also have formed organizations. These organizations and the pathways to specialty certification differ from their American counterparts. A number of examples of national and international collaboration between psychiatric organizations leading to positive outcomes can be cited.

PSYCHIATRIC CLINICS
OF NORTH AMERICA

FORTHCOMING ISSUES

June 2008

Suicidal Behavior: A Developmental Perspective
J. John Mann, MD and Maria Oquendo, MD,
Guest Editors

September 2008

Personality Disorders
Joel Paris, MD, *Guest Editor*

RECENT ISSUES

December 2007

Psychosomatic Medicine
James L. Levenson, MD, David F. Gitlin, MD, and
Cathy Crone, MD, *Guest Editors*

September 2007

**Schizophrenia: A Complex Disease
Necessitating Complex Care**
Peter F. Buckley, MD and Erick L. Messias, MD, MPH, PhD,
Guest Editors

June 2007

Clinical Interviewing: Practical Tips from Master Clinicians
Shawn Christopher Shea, MD,
Guest Editor

Psychiatr Clin N Am 31 (2008) xiii–xv

PSYCHIATRIC CLINICS
OF NORTH AMERICA

Preface

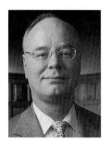
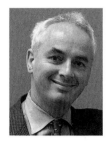

Daniel R. Wilson, MD, PhD
Peter F. Buckley, MD

Guest Editors

P sychiatry is not merely a branch of general medicine–it has a history and present configuration that is otherwise totally unique in medicine. Yet in the past 50 years the scope of psychiatry has moved far beyond the old institutional basis even as it is ever more enriched by developments in general medicine, technology, and systems of care. Indeed, the science of psychiatry is in a golden age of great accumulating insight into genes, brains, and minds all so much in the literature.

Yet psychiatry is tarnished and eroded by a host of political, economic, and social troubles. Still, there is much reason for optimism as this unique field begins to move toward a stronger foundation in knowledge while addressing many stubborn problems in finance, administration, and the integration of new science with novel systems of care.

This issue of the *Psychiatric Clinics of North America* surveys not the "content" of psychiatric sciences but the "processes" by which the care of millions of suffering human beings is being dramatically reshaped despite many setbacks, generally for the better. These diverse qualitative and technical developments touch the individual practitioner and affect every component of the health system with increasing benefit to the care of patients and society at large.

In "Transforming Mental Health Care: Realities, Priorities, and Prospects," Hogan–one of the nation's most senior mental health administrators and Chair of the President's New Freedom Commission–offers a crisp summary of the state of play in and predictions about mental health care. Key trends, threats and opportunities are identified as they affect every element and every practitioner in the "system." In his article "Financing Mental Health and Substance Use Disorder Care Within Physical Health: A Look to the Future," Kathol, an

0193-953X/08/$ – see front matter
doi:10.1016/j.psc.2008.01.001

internist-psychiatrist who has pioneered systems of more integrated care, explains critical issues and new directions of behavioral health care delivery and investment. Essential problems and solutions for societal investment in psychiatric care are summarized.

Tesar reviews the history of and prospects for hospital and academic psychiatry from his perspective as Chief of Psychiatry at the Cleveland Clinic. "Whither Hospital and Academic Psychiatry?" is a thoughtful and substantive review of how things came to be as they are and where they may be headed. In "Applying the Institute of Medicine Quality Chasm Framework to Improving Health Care for Mental and Substance Use Conditions," Keyser and colleagues summarize the basic themes of quality enhancement, an increasingly common focus of modern medicine. This group of experts further clarifies how such a focus will likely impact psychiatry.

In "Quality Outcomes Management: Veterans Affairs Case Study," Bhatia and Fernandes offer a clear example of quality enhancement, which has so remarkably advanced care within the Veterans' heath system. This report from the front lines of care management explains how the largest health care system in the United States has implemented a wide range of technologic and service delivery improvements. Compton skillfully surveys the important but too easily neglected topic of prevention in mental health in "Incorporating the Prevention Paradigm into Administrative Psychiatry." Here the effort is to mitigate risk factors and enhance protective factors and thereby decrease the burden of psychiatric illness.

In "Telepsychiatry Reduces Geographic Physician Disparity in Rural Settings, But Is It Financially Feasible Because of Reimbursement?" Hilty and colleagues examine the current state and potential of technology to improve patient access to appropriate mental health services across disparate geography and populations. Noting the clear feasibility of such services, they also caution that several administrative and financial impediments must yet be overcome. Lawlor and Barrows summarize the promise and problems associated with electronic health records as experienced in psychiatry in "Behavioral Health Electronic Medical Record." Like telepsychiatry, they note the eventual use of such records once administrative and financial impediments are addressed.

In "Leadership and Professional Workforce Development," Buckley and Madaan provide a brief review on how recruitment into psychiatry has been cyclical and shaped by major developments in psychiatric practice, teaching, and other societal issues. After tracing the history and current conditions of professional workforce development, they lay out several important points for further success in the future. Scheiber and colleagues provide a historical overview of the ABPN; its formation, mission, and roles; and the changes that have taken place over the years in certification, recertification, and maintenance of the certification process.

Finally, in "Psychiatry: Organized and Disorganized," Munro and Wilson describe psychiatry as a specialty with an array of clinical, research, and didactic responsibilities that span a range of social, economic, political, and administrative interests broader than that of any other medical specialty. They further survey the depth and breadth of how psychiatry is organized (or not), all as reflected in the complex tapestry woven by its varied constituent organizations.

Daniel R. Wilson, MD, PhD
Professor and Chairman of Psychiatry
Professor of Anthropology
Creighton University Medical Center
3528 Dodge Street, Omaha, NE 68131 USA

E-mail address: wilson@creighton.edu

Peter F. Buckley, MD
Professor and Chairman, Department of Psychiatry and Health Behavior
Medical College of Georgia
1515 Pope Avenue
Augusta, GA 30912-3800

E-mail address: pbuckley@mail.mcg.edu

Psychiatr Clin N Am 31 (2008) 1–9

PSYCHIATRIC CLINICS
OF NORTH AMERICA

Transforming Mental Health Care: Realities, Priorities, and Prospects

Michael F. Hogan, PhD

New York State Office of Mental Health, 44 Holland Avenue, Albany, NY 12229, USA

The past two decades have placed mental health in the national spotlight in areas ranging from research (the National Institute on Mental Health's "Decade of the Brain") to political and policy visibility (the Clinton Administration's White House Conference on Mental Health, the nation's first Surgeon General's Report on Mental Health [1], and the President's New Freedom Commission on Mental Health [2]). Changes in patterns of care were also significant. The release of Prozac and the bevy of other safer, easy-to-prescribe treatments for depression that followed it doubled the treated prevalence of this common and often disabling illness [3]. A host of new treatments for psychotic illnesses (the second-generation or atypical antipsychotics) led to dramatic shifts in patterns of treatment for these conditions. One might conclude that mental illness is finally emerging from the shadows, and that the benefits of scientific progress, improvements in treatment, and improved mental health policy have finally changed the paradigm of brain disorders as chronic conditions treated in a second-class specialty system.

To borrow a phrase from the economic debate of this same period, this conclusion may well be characterized as "irrational exuberance." Although advances occurred, those with the most serious mental illness (SMI) continue to struggle. Examples include the incarceration of people with mental illness, the worsening affordability of housing, and new evidence about the premature mortality of people with mental illness [4]. Which view of trends in mental health is more accurate, boom or bust? To the extent trends can be seen, what forces are shaping them? In this muddled context, what are the prospects for the "transformation" of mental health care called for by the President's Commission?

It is probably too early to judge the impact of this commission. A remarkable new analysis of mental health policy, however, provides a lucid perspective on the status and impact of changes in mental health. The monograph *Better but not well: mental health policy in the United States since 1950* is a systematic attempt to answer two questions: are people with a mental illness better off today than

E-mail address: Cocomfh@omh.state.ny.us

0193-953X/08/$ – see front matter
doi:10.1016/j.psc.2007.12.001

a generation ago, and if so why? Frank and Glied [5] have created a framework to evaluate needs and prospects for change in mental health care. This article considers their analysis and the prospects for transforming mental health care.

THE WELL-BEING OF PEOPLE WITH A MENTAL ILLNESS

Frank and Glied [5] assess the status of people with mental illness by comparing data from dozens of national sources over the period, covering such topics as the prevalence and treated prevalence of those with mental illness to the quality of available and provided treatments, to housing and income status, to the cost of care. The picture that emerges is, overall, one of progress. Quoting President Kennedy's 1963 message to the US Congress, Frank and Glied [5] conclude "The nation has made notable progress toward nearly all the goals he articulated in 1963. The lives of people with mental disorders are much more similar to those of most Americans today than they were in 1960. The material lives of the majority of people with these conditions are measurably improved."

The path to and patterns of improvement manifested over the years is not, however, what President Kennedy or his advisors envisioned: a focus on an improved mental health system and on therapeutic advances. This strategy of "exceptionalism" has been less fruitful than what Frank and Glied [5] term a "mainstreaming" strategy by which people with mental illness benefit from improvements in general social welfare and health programs. Indeed, the improvement in these benefits over the past generation has been remarkable. At the time of President Kennedy's speech, Medicare, Medicaid, Supplemental Security Income (SSI), and Social Security Disability Income did not exist. Private health insurance was available to far fewer people, and it often had limited if any benefits for medications (the major treatment modality for most mental illness) or for mental health interventions, such as psychotherapy.

Covering all of these trends in detail is beyond the scope of this article, and Frank and Glied [5] have done it exceptionally well. Yet, even the mention of the programs listed previously gives a good sense of their impact on those with a mental illness. What can be said about the contribution of mental health services, and from the explosion in research over this period? Several examples illustrate the limits of change in this arena: one focused on specialty mental health policy and one focused on improvements in treatment technology.

In the services arena, the history and impact of the community mental health centers program illustrates the limits of reforms focused on improving mental health care. It is a useful cautionary tale because the community mental health centers program was a core strategy proposed by President Kennedy. Originally hoped to lead to community mental health centers in every community, the program was first limited by a 7-year time cap on funding. Growth of the program then fell victim to budget pressures and competition. Finally, it was converted into a block grant during the Reagan years. Today, the mental health block grant totals about $430 million, less than the mental health budgets of over a dozen states, and the block grant allocation to many states is less than 1% of their overall mental health budget [6]. Gronfein [7] compared the impact of the community mental health centers program on mental health care with that of Medicaid. He found that community mental health centers did contribute to reduced levels of state hospitalization, but the impact was far less than Medicaid's. Additionally, although Medicaid contributed to increased state mental health spending (affecting overall state policy), the community mental health centers program did not similarly contribute.

Another example of the less-than-anticipated impact of specialty mental health care is the impact of innovation in generating new and more effective treatments. The case of treatments for schizophrenia offers a cautionary tale. How much more efficacious are the treatments, both drugs and other therapies, than those available a generation ago? During the 1990s, the second-generation or atypical antipsychotics were introduced with great fanfare, promising greater symptom relief and reduced side effects. Billions of dollars later, as these medicines start to go off patent, it is now evident that the promised increased efficacy of these treatments was greatly exaggerated, whereas the pattern of side effects including weight gain and risk of diabetes is probably comparable with the side effect risks of the older drugs [8].

These examples illustrate the limits of advancing outcomes and experiences for people with mental illness solely within the mental health system, and the importance of advocacy strategies that improve health and social insurance programs. There is also work to be done to tailor these benefits to the particular needs of those with mental illness. This perspective does not render insignificant the tasks of managing and providing good mental health care. Given the substantial but incomplete progress achieved over the last generation, what strategies are needed and relevant today, especially for clinicians and advocates focused on the well-being of those with SMI?

THE CHALLENGE OF TRANSFORMING MENTAL HEALTH CARE

Accepting that the well-being of those with mental illness has been most affected by improvements in mainstream benefits scarcely implies that work to improve mental health care itself is unnecessary or impossible. This is illustrated by comparisons at every level of care. From the clinical level (eg, comparing the impact of good versus bad treatment on the outcomes that individuals achieve) to a systems view (eg, the comparisons of state systems periodically conducted by the National Alliance on Mental Illness [9]) it is evident that quality makes a difference even if it is hard to define. (The challenges of defining quality of care bring to mind the famous quote from Supreme Court Justice Potter Stewart that pornography is hard to define "but I know it when I see it" [10].)

Fragmented Care as A Target of Reform

Care for adults or children with SMI is very complex (for many individuals involving elements of medical illness, psychologic difficulty, trauma, poverty, disability, and an uneven and often prolonged course). Achieving good care requires orchestrating programs and bureaucracies that address all of these challenges in a fashion that meets individual needs, in a complex interagency and multilevel political environment. The differentiation of the systems and political environment leads to fragmented care. These complexities help explain, as Grob and Goldman [11] have noted, why broad reviews of mental health care, such as both the Carter Commission [12] and the Bush-appointed New Freedom Commission, focus on the fragmentation of care as a core problem. "Fragmentation" is easy to comprehend; "falling through the cracks" has become part of the vernacular, and public awareness of the complexity of the health and behavioral health systems creates a fertile understanding for these images.

The challenge of solving this problem is much more complex. Diagnoses of systems failure like "fragmentation" (and solutions like "services integration" or "transformation") are evocative but not very concrete. These descriptions are more metaphor than theory, and they have diffuse connotations. Decades ago, over two dozen strategies to achieve coordination were identified [13]. Part of the problem in addressing this problem is that solutions cut across jurisdictional boundaries that are enforced by legislative bodies, spurred on by affected constituencies. Fragmentation of interests leads indirectly to fragmentation of services. This observation led Marmor and Gill [14] to suggest that comprehensive mental health reform is unlikely in the United States, because "the political system places fundamental constraints on the mobilization of resources to solve the profound needs of the mental health care delivery system." The fragmentation of care remains a serious problem, but one that is extremely hard to address in any systematic fashion.

Other Major Challenges for Transforming Care

What then are other major challenges for the well-being of people with SMI that demand attention, and are perhaps less diffuse than fragmented care? This analysis considers two recent national reviews (Frank and Glied's [5] assessment and the report of the presidential commission). It focuses on major problems where steps can be taken both by improving or refocusing mental health care, and also by achieving changes or accommodations in mainstream programs that are essential if they are adequately to serve the substantial population of individuals with SMI. The list of "transformation targets" that follows is not definitive; other challenges might easily be substituted. The following brief list includes several substantial problems that can be, and must be, addressed both by improvements in specialty mental health care and by making adjustments in mainstream programs:

1. The poor employment status and resultant poverty of people with SMI that has persisted despite improved benefits
2. The eroding supply of affordable housing on which people with SMI depend
3. The delayed diagnosis and access to care for children with mental disorders
4. An epidemic of comorbid chronic physical illnesses among those with SMI

Discussed next is the case for the significance of these problems and prospects for change.

POOR EMPLOYMENT STATUS AND RESULTANT POVERTY

Although a focus on employment is often outside the scope of treatment, partly because of this, a strong case can be made that unemployment is the most substantial problem for people with SMI. Although people with mental illness consistently express strong and realistic preferences to get a job, workforce participation levels are lower for people with a mental illness than for those with any other illness-related disability, people with mental illness are the largest and fastest growing group on SSI, and people with mental illness are both the largest disability group entering the vocational rehabilitation system and the group with the worst outcomes [15]. The low rate of employment, coupled with relatively stingy social welfare benefits in the United States compared with Western Europe, is the major reason why most individuals with SMI live below the poverty level [5]. What are the major reasons for this state of affairs, and what can be done to address it?

A general lack of attention to employment concerns within the mental health system is certainly a major culprit, and one that can be remedied by leadership. Substantial progress on increasing employment levels requires two major strategies, however, each requiring adaptation of major federal programs to the needs of people with SMI and leadership in states and communities.

The first strategy is to make the effective and evidence-based approach of supported employment available on a widespread, near-universal basis for people with SMI. In multiple studies, supported employment has shown both superior effectiveness over other approaches and its implementability without unrealistic staff requirements [16]. The difficulty is that supported employment methods effective for people with supported employment are not accommodated well by the federally supported vocational rehabilitation program, whereas employment supports are not a covered service under Medicaid, which has become the major payer for mental health care. Additionally, the disincentives to employment in Social Security (especially the threat of lost Medicaid eligibility) are strong. Programs to address these disincentives are complex and arcane, and little used. Unless adjustments to vocational rehabilitation and Medicaid are made to reimburse better for supported employment (making it feasible in most communities) and Social Security creates better ways to ameliorate disincentives, the tragic unemployment of people with SMI will continue. These changes (a focus on employment with mental health programs and systems, and targeted reform of these federal programs so they better meet the needs of the SMI population) are urgent next steps to help consumers achieve employment and the benefits it affords.

ERODING ACCESS TO AFFORDABLE HOUSING

Frank and Glied [5] cite the expansion of the Section 8 housing subsidy program among the mainstream benefit expansions that have benefited those with a mental illness. The scaled-back federal role in low-income housing production, rising levels of low-income housing affordability, and static levels of Section 8 subsidies have together created a worsening national environment for the housing that most people with SMI rely on. Nationally, O'Hara and colleagues [17] report that the rental price of the average one-bedroom apartment (which cost 86% of the average monthly SSI subsidy in 1998) by 2006 cost 114% of this benefit. People with SMI are priced out of the housing marketplace.

To respond, many state mental health authorities have developed programs to build and finance housing for people with SMI. The New York State Office of Mental Health, one of the leaders in this area, by 2007 had 39,000 units of housing (including residential services, such as group homes) dedicated to people with SMI in place or in the construction-renovation pipeline. This included a commitment of over $200 million for new housing in the 2007 to 2008 budget alone. The scope of the problem dwarfs this solution, however, and few states have developed housing as aggressively as New York. With about 250,000 SMI individuals in New York State reliant on SSI income, a generally worsening low-income housing marketplace, and increased competition for available units (eg, from state prisoners reaching the end of their sentences and re-entering local communities), the housing crunch is too massive to be met by development of specialized "mental health housing."

Although multiple housing development strategies should be used within the mental health world [18], the housing challenge cannot be met without federal leadership. Whether by tax incentives, expanded rental subsidies, an increase in SSI, or a renewed federal commitment for development of additional units, federal resources must be brought to bear on the problem of affordable housing for poor people with disabilities, especially those with SMI. This issue requires a mixture of actions within the mental health system, and collaboration with housing advocates on national strategies.

LATE DIAGNOSIS AND ACCESS TO CARE FOR CHILDREN

Since Burns and colleagues [19] reported that only one of five youth with mental disorders are seen or treated by mental health specialists, this systemic problem has been well known. With the results of the National Co-morbidity Study Replication the scope of the problem is even more evident. First, it is now more apparent that the onset of most mental illness is in adolescence, with a median age of onset under 14 years. Second, the delays in accessing care are extraordinary, with waits of over 10 years from earliest symptoms to first entry into care more the rule than the exception [20].

This problem is exacerbated by the national shortage of child psychiatrists [21]. Adequate, systematic solutions to the problem are lacking. The numbers of child psychiatrists in training is not increasing, and the "rate-limiting factors" that constrain the supply of child psychiatrists (eg, additional required year of training, shortage of mentors, challenging practice conditions, and relatively low compensation) are potent. Pediatricians already provide most mental health care for children, but in many cases are inadequately trained or compensated for this work.

Robust solutions to the problem of late entry into care may be lacking, but many approaches are being designed and implemented. These include efforts to align pediatrics and psychiatry; increased school health and mental health programs; and New York State's Child and Family Clinic Plus program, which deploys child clinicians to "settings where the children are," such as schools, child welfare settings, and pediatric practices. Improvements within the mental health system are necessary (eg, deploying child specialists to schools and pediatric settings). In the broader arena, increased attention to child mental health in mainstream settings must occur. Accommodations must recognize the scope of the problem and take tangible steps to address the problem (eg, compensation for pediatricians that recognizes the complexity of diagnosing and treating mental disorders).

THE EPIDEMIC OF COMORBID CHRONIC PHYSICAL ILLNESSES AMONG THOSE WITH SERIOUS MENTAL ILLNESS

The term "epidemic" is now used routinely to describe the escalating prevalence of diabetes in the United States; the trend follows patterns of increased obesity. Perhaps in part because of attention to this issue, and perhaps because of awareness of the weight gain associated with many of the newer antipsychotic agents, premature mortality associated with physical illnesses among those with SMI has received recent attention. The medical directors of the state mental health agencies summarized these problems in a recent monograph [4]. They found that a number of recent studies have documented high rates of premature death (25–30 years on average) for SMI individuals, with cardiac illness and diabetes being the major causes of premature death. These high death rates for a population under care are a compelling call to action.

Because of the urgency of the problem and because underlying trends (eg, obesity) in the general population are worsening, the problem of premature death demands increased attention. This is also a problem that must be addressed through broad public health measures and health care that is preventive, but also one that requires action in mental health circles. Although the well-established pattern of people with SMI getting poor care in mainstream health settings must be addressed, mental health settings must also attend to and provide wellness-oriented primary care services. There are many actions that should be taken in mental health clinics, day programs, and rehabilitation settings to attack the problem: monitoring of weight, waist circumference, or body mass index; smoking cessation programs; ensuring that people with SMI receive convenient general medical care; and orienting care to a goal of overall wellness, not just recovery from mental illness.

SUMMARY

Mental health care is emerging from a period of remarkable, if possibly evanescent, national attention. The Decade of the Brain, the first White House conference and Surgeon General's reports on mental health, and the first presidential commission in a generation to focus on this area indicate that concern about mental health is rising. At the same time, many old problems remain. A long view finds that the circumstances of people with a mental illness are "better but not well" [5] and that advances and efforts specific to mental health have contributed less than have incremental improvements in mainstream programs, such as Medicaid and Medicare.

The next stage of improving the well-being of people with SMI must be informed by what has been learned about the nature of the problems, and also about the solutions that work. There is much to be done to address the challenges that remain within mental health settings. As much as the rising tide of improved general benefits has benefited people with SMI, their well-being remains marginal, and tailored adjustments to these mainstream programs are essential. The national attention on mental health issues seen in the last decade has been pleasant, but experience suggests that "big bang" change is unlikely to result. Instead, transforming mental health care requires focused work on midrange challenges, if recovery and wellness are to be made the expected reality for people with mental illness.

References

[1] US Department of Health and Human Services. Mental health: a report of the Surgeon General. Rockville (MD): U.S. Department of Health and Human Services, Substance Abuse and Mental Health Services Administration, Center for Mental Health Services, National Institutes of Health, National Institute of Mental Health; 1999.

[2] New Freedom Commission on Mental Health. Achieving the promise: transforming mental health care in America final report. Rockville (MD): DHHS; Pub. NO. SMA-03-3832 2003.

[3] Wang PS, Demler O, Olfson M, et al. Changing profiles of service sectors used for mental health care in the US. Am J Psychiatry 2006;163(7):1187–98.

[4] National Association of State Mental Health Program Directors. Morbidity and mortality in People with Serious Mental Illness Technical Report. Alexandria (VA): 2006.

[5] Frank RG, Glied SA. Better but not well: mental health policy in the United States since 1950. Baltimore (MD): John Hopkins, University Press; 2006.

[6] Lutterman T. Fiscal year 2005 state mental health agency revenues and expenditures. Alexandria (VA): National Association of State Mental Health Program Directors Research Institute; in press.

[7] Gronfein W. Incentives and intentions in mental health policy: a comparison of the Medicaid and community mental health programs. J Health Soc Behav 1995;26:192–206.

[8] McEvoy JP, Meyer JM, Goff DC, et al. Prevalence of the metabolic syndrome in patients with schizophrenia: baseline results from the Clinical Antipsychotic Trials of Intervention Effectiveness (CATIE), schizophrenia trial and comparison with national estimates from the NHANES III. Schizophr Res 2005;80:90–132.

[9] National Alliance on Mental Illness. Grading the states: a report of America's health care system for serious mental illness. Alexandria (VA): National Alliance on Mental Illness; 2006.

[10] Jacobelis v. Ohio (1964). 378 U.S. 184.

[11] Grob GN, Goldman HH. The dilemma of federal mental health policy: radical reform or incremental change?. Brunswick (NJ): Rutgers's University Press; 2006.

[12] U.S. President's Commission on Mental Health. Report to the President from the President's Commission on Mental Health. Washington, DC: U.S. Government Printing Office; 1978.

[13] Hogan M, MacEachron AE. Plan evaluation guide: a guide to the planning, management and evaluation of community-based service systems. Toronto: National Institute on Mental Retardation; 1980.

[14] Marmor TR, Gill KC. The political and economic context of mental health care in the United States. J Health Polit Policy Law 1989;15:459–75.
[15] New Freedom Commission on Mental Health. Interim report of the President's New Freedom Commission on Mental Health. 2002 Available at: http://mentalhealthcommission.gov/reports/Interim_Report.htm. Accessed November 1, 2007.
[16] Bond GR. Supported employment: evidence for evidence-based practice. Psychiatr Rehabil J 2004;27:345–59.
[17] O'Hara A, Cooper E, Zovistoski A, et al. Priced out in 2006: the housing crisis for people with disabilities. Boston: Technical Assistance Collaborative; 2007.
[18] O'Hara A. Housing for people with mental illness: update of a report to the President's New Freedom Commission. Psychiatr Serv 2007;58:907–13.
[19] Burns BJ, Costello EJ, Angold A, et al. Children's mental health services use across service sectors. Health Aff 1995;14:147–59.
[20] Wang PS, Berglund P, Olfson M, et al. Failure and delay in initial treatment contact after first onset of mental disorders in the National Co-morbidity Survey Replication. Arch Gen Psychiatry 2005;62(6):603–13.
[21] Thomas CR, Holzer CE. The continuing shortage of child and adolescent psychiatrists. J Am Acad Child Adolesc Psychiatry 2006;45(9):1023–31.

Financing Mental Health and Substance Use Disorder Care Within Physical Health: A Look to the Future

Roger G. Kathol, MD[a,b,c,*], Steve Melek, BA[d], Byron Bair, MD[e,f], Susan Sargent, MBA[g]

[a]Department of Medicine, University of Minnesota Medical School, 420 Delaware Street SE, MMC 194, Suite 14-106 Phillips-Wangensteen Building, Minneapolis, MN 55455, USA
[b]Department of Psychiatry, University of Minnesota Medical School, F282/2A West, 2450 Riverside Avenue South, Minneapolis, MN 55454, USA
[c]Cartesian Solutions, Inc., 3004 Foxpoint Road, Burnsville, MN 55337, USA
[d]Milliman, Inc., 1099 18th Street, Suite 3100, Denver, CO 80202, USA
[e]University of Utah School of Medicine, 50 N Medical Drive, Room 4B120 Salt Lake City, UT 84132, USA
[f]Salt Lake City Veterans Administration Hospital, 500 Foothill Boulevard, Salt Lake City, UT 84148, USA
[g]Array Healthcare Facilities Solutions, 2520 Renaissance Boulevard, Suite 110, King of Prussia, PA 19406, USA

There is a major and illogical dichotomy in the systems for providing and for financing medical and psychiatric care. Ninety percent of patients who have mental health/substance use disorders (MH/SUDs) are seen in the general medical sector, but the entire focus in the distribution of MH/SUDs health-related resources, with the exception of payment for psychotropic medications, is on the 10% seen exclusively in the mental health sector [1,2]. Even in the specialty sector, only about half of patients who have MH/SUDs receive minimally adequate care. Two thirds of patients who have MH/SUDs seen in general medicine receive no treatment for their behavioral illnesses, and, of the third who are treated, only one tenth receive evidence-based approaches to care [2–4]. This situation results in patients who have MH/SUDs using twice as many total health care resources (80% of which are for medical tests, procedures, and medications), having worse physical and mental health outcomes, and suffering greater impairment than those without these disorders [5,6].

Meanwhile, national spending trends for MH/SUDs during the last 2 decades have been remarkable. Prescription drug costs for MH/SUDs have

*Corresponding author. Cartesian Solutions, Inc., 3004 Foxpoint Road, Burnsville, MN 55337. E-mail address: roger-kathol@cartesiansolutions.com (R.G. Kathol).

0193-953X/08/$ – see front matter
doi:10.1016/j.psc.2007.11.001

risen rapidly, from just 7% of total mental health spending in 1986 to 23% in 2003. They are projected to account for 30% of all mental health spending by 2014. Total hospital costs (including inpatient acute services and outpatient services such as day treatment) dropped from 41% in 1986 to 28% of total mental health spending in 2003 while physician services increased from 11% in 1986 to 14% in 2003.

Even the 10% of psychiatric patients seen in MH/SUD settings receive inferior care because a high percentage have concurrent physical health problems. Living in a segregated medical system, they have trouble receiving general medical services coordinated with their MH/SUD care because of the separation of medical and psychiatric records, isolated service locations, and the disconnection of MH/SUD from physical health clinicians [7]. In today's health care environment, MH/SUD and physical health professionals have little organizational incentive to communicate and do not feel accountable for cross-disciplinary outcomes in the common patients they serve. As a result of this lack of interaction between general medical and psychiatric care, outcomes suffer, costs escalate, and patients die much earlier than their non–mentally ill counterparts [5,8].

Psychiatric administrators often consider the separation of dollars dedicated to general medical and mental health care necessary to preserve adequate support for patients who have behavioral disorders. On almost every front, this misconception flies in the face of the evidence. As already mentioned, 60% of patients receive no MH/SUD treatment at all. Another 32% get clearly inadequate treatment, leaving a mere 8% of patients who have MH/SUDs receiving minimally adequate care today in the United States. These statistics suggest that the independence of behavioral health dollars has done little to support MH/SUD treatment for most patients.

Even patients seen in the MH/SUD sector have not fared well. The value of the health care dollars spent for MH/SUD care dropped by 54% between 1988 and 1998, fourfold greater than the loss in value of dollars spent for general medical care [9]. This change occurred at a time when behavioral health advocates were independently and aggressively arguing for the needs of their patients who had MH/SUD. Further, many of the most complex and costly patients who have MH/SUDs seen in the behavioral sector have concurrent physical illness, but separate reimbursement business practices prevent practitioners from knowing that cross-disciplinary care is needed or being given. In such an environment, there is not even an opportunity to improve cost and outcomes, because physical and MH/SUD care practitioners are working blindly with each other's patients. There is no coordination or collaboration [10].

The picture painted here is not pretty, but initial steps are being taken to overcome the barriers to effective treatment faced by patients who have MH/SUDs. This article describes the important interaction between general medical and psychiatric illness, discusses early steps being taken to improve evidence-based service access and outcomes for patients who have psychiatric illness, most of whom are seen in the primary care setting, and defines the next steps required for transforming the present situation.

CASE SCENARIOS
Mr. S

Mr. S came to the emergency room with acute right lower quadrant abdominal pain. A diagnosis of appendicitis was made. Routine laboratory examinations were unremarkable. Routine surgical preoperative preparations were completed, and Mr. S's appendix was removed successfully within 8 hours of his arrival at the emergency room.

Postoperatively, Mr. S developed symptoms of hypertension, tachycardia, and episodes of visual hallucinations. Discussions with his wife revealed that Mr. S had been drinking several beers each day for the past several months to treat what his wife described as intense anxiety, lack of energy, and feelings of depression. Alcohol withdrawal was diagnosed, and treatment initiated. As a result of agitation during alcohol withdrawal, Mr. S's surgical wound dehisced. He developed a wound infection and aspirated while fighting his restraints. Pneumonia ensued with respiratory compromise requiring intubation and an ICU stay of 1 week. After a prolonged hospitalization related to complications, he was discharged to an extended-care facility for rehabilitation. Underlying issues of his alcohol dependence, anxiety, and depression were never addressed by the treatment teams while he was hospitalized.

Ms R

Ms R had been seeing Dr. X for several years for thyroid disorder and hypertension. During the past 3 years she had multiple persistent symptoms that included difficulty sleeping, intermittent feelings she was about to pass out, sharp chest pain, fatigue, and difficulty focusing on routine tasks. Because of these symptoms, she stopped doing many of the things that she enjoyed. Her primary care physician had performed many medical evaluations to find the cause, including stress EKGs, a multiple-gated acquisition scan, and even cardiac catheterization. She denied having problems with depression but was never asked about symptoms compatible with it.

Consultations with many of the specialists within the group practice were made including cardiology, neurology, infectious disease, endocrinology, and rheumatology. None proved beneficial. She was going to the emergency room an average of one to two times per month. Her primary care provider was becoming increasingly frustrated with her visits, because every avenue explored seemed fruitless.

During a recent appointment, Ms R reported that if nothing could be done to treat her symptoms, she would be "better off dead." This statement prompted her doctor to place an emergent consult to psychiatry. Ms. R was incensed by this action, stated that she would never come back to Dr. X's office again, and left the office threatening him with a lawsuit. That afternoon, she went to the local emergency room complaining of being faint and dizzy and demanded to be hospitalized on the medical surgical floor until her symptoms could be diagnosed and managed. She refused to leave the emergency room until she received the treatment she expected.

Mr. T

Mr. T had been diagnosed as having schizoaffective disorder and had been seen regularly in the local community mental health center. His symptoms were controlled with a combination of antidepressant, anticonvulsant, and antipsychotic medications. Whenever he had a medical problem, he would go to an urgent care center. These visits were prompted by some type of respiratory complaint and were fairly infrequent.

His psychiatric condition had been stable for several years, and there were no obvious side effects from his medications, such as obesity or excess sedation. Over the past few visits, Mr. T complained that he had to urinate more frequently, and he wondered if his bladder was infested with alien life forms. His antipsychotic dose was increased without positive effects. One afternoon, Mr. T failed to show up to his regularly scheduled mental health appointment. A social worker called his home, and Mr. T answered but had slurred speech. An ambulance was sent to Mr. T's house where he was found very confused, hypotensive, and lethargic. He was taken to the emergency room where he was evaluated.

Mr. T was severely dehydrated, and his blood glucose level was 750 mg/dL. He was hospitalized for diabetic hyperosmolar coma. The medical record revealed that Mr. T had not had a blood chemistry done for more than 10 years. There also were no records of immunizations or routine medical evaluations. During his hospitalization, it was discovered that Mr. T also had hypothyroidism, hypertension, hyperlipidemia, and severe iron deficiency anemia, as well as type II diabetes mellitus. It was unclear what role his psychiatric medications played in his current medical condition, because there were no previous medical records.

In case his antipsychotic medication had contributed to the endocrinology disorders, his psychiatric medications were either decreased or discontinued, prompting an acute exacerbation of his underlying schizoaffective disorder. His behavior was uncontrollable in the hospital and prevented treatment of his underlying medical conditions. He was given intravenous sedation, which controlled his hyperactivity, but he became overly sedated, aspirated, and had an acute respiratory arrest. He could not be resuscitated successfully, and he died after 3 weeks in the hospital.

ADVANCING QUALITY CARE THROUGH REVISED FUNDING ARRANGEMENTS FOR BEHAVIORAL HEALTH

Mental health clinicians strive valiantly to reverse suffering among those who have MH/SUDs, but the reimbursement environment forces them to work apart from all other health practitioners under guidelines that focus more on the number of interventions per year than on holistic patient outcomes that integrate mental and physical health parameters. As long as MH/SUD service support remains segregated, costs for physical health services in patients who have MH/SUDs will continue to shift from the behavioral health sector to the physical health sector. Moreover, costs will rise, and overall clinical improvement will be limited [11].

A small but growing number of forward-thinking health care delivery systems are beginning to recognize the important contribution that MH/SUD care plays in the success of physical health treatment, especially in patients who have chronic and/or acute but serious medical conditions. As a result, these organizations view MH/SUD care as an integral part of health and include MH/SUD providers and facilities in contract negotiations, not as stand-alone entities with separate payment arrangements but as core components of the health delivery process.

Such an altered perspective allows the creation of clinical settings with MH/SUD and physical health practitioners working side by side in both primary care settings and MH/SUD clinics. It facilitates the creation and supports the operation of inpatient clinical settings (ie, medical psychiatry units) in which patients who have comorbid general medical and psychiatric illness can receive aggressive, evidence-based interventions for all types of illnesses from the first day of hospitalization. It allows the institution of inpatient, outpatient, and continued care programs, such as delirium prevention programs, primary care–based buprenorphine clinics, and integrated general medical and behavioral geriatric programs, that lead to improved quality of care, lowered impairment, and reduced total health care costs [5].

Compelling evidence shows that untreated or ineffectively treated patients who have MH/SUDs–with or without concurrent general medical illness–manifest persistent complexity and high use of general medical health services [6]. Seeing the benefits of integrated care, general medical health plans are becoming more responsive to requests to consolidate reimbursement for MH/SUD care with physical health care. By supporting better MH/SUD care in all clinical settings, they reason, they will be able to reduce the high cost of care shifted to physical health benefits [11].

REIMBURSEMENT FOR MENTAL HEALTH/SUBSTANCE USE DISORDER SERVICES AS A PART OF PHYSICAL HEALTH BENEFITS

In the past 5 years, numerous general medical health plans (eg, Aetna, Humana, Amerigroup, and Blue Cross/Blue Shield of Massachusetts, just to name a few) have insourced their behavioral health business. This insourcing is the first step in a growing trend by health plans to integrate MH/SUD with physical health care benefits in response to demands by both commercial and public program clients. This integration cannot be done when MH/SUDs are managed independently, as through a behavioral health carve-out. To date, most of the health plans that have taken this step continue to use separate MH/SUD care business practices, as if the business were carved out [5]. Thus, little advantage is realized by either patients or the health plan. Insourced

MH/SUD responsibility that lacks integrated business practices is known as "carved-in" behavioral health. Nonetheless, insourcing MH/SUD business provides general medical health plans with an ability to consider innovative contract arrangements not possible when the MH/SUD business is owned by an external vendor. Increasingly, such contract alterations are being considered. In a small but growing number of plans, they are being implemented.

One of the first areas in which this is taking place is through support for "integrated" case and disease management for patients who have physical and MH/SUDs. Case and disease management are designed to assist clinicians with chronic and/or complex patients by helping the patients overcome barriers to improvement, such as understanding their illnesses, filling prescriptions, showing up for appointments, coordinating communication among treating physicians, and finding transportation to tests and appointments. When care management is integrated, issues related to both medical and psychiatric disorders are addressed. This assistance can occur onsite in clinic settings that treat patients who have highly complex conditions; it can be performed by telephone from a central offsite location; or it can be provided via Web-based systems integrated with the electronic medical record, as in the Veterans Administration demonstration Care Coordination projects.

Actuarial projections for integrated case and disease management suggest that augmented clinical outcomes for patients will lead to substantially lower long-term total health care costs, as well as other reduced costs to employers, and to a healthier population. For example, an analysis of the impact such integration could have on the employer's health care costs, sick day costs, disability costs, and productivity levels was completed for a large self-insured group. This projection showed that an employer of 31,400 workers could save about $3 million per year by the successful integration of medical and behavioral health care services.

The more forward-thinking general medical health plans that have insourced their behavioral health business now are also initiating steps to integrate care at the clinical level. This change is made through the use of altered patient and provider contract terminology that can support the integration of general medical and psychiatric service delivery, regardless of location. Although case and disease management can help patients adhere to clinicians' recommendations, such management cannot alter the fragmentation of general medical and behavioral health services available to patients. These health plans are adding value through contract language that allows hospitals and clinics to establish financially solvent, colocated clinical services. These services include primary care clinics with onsite MH/SUD personnel as a part of the medical team, proactive general hospital emergency room and inpatient psychiatric consultation services, medical psychiatry units, and delirium prevention programs.

General medical health plans that have insourced behavioral health business also are poised to take advantage of other economies potentially associated with care for the whole patient. All clinicians, including MH/SUD professionals, can be included in the general medical health plan provider networks.

Quality improvement programs can include work process changes that support coordinated physical and MH/SUD care. Coding and billing procedures can be consolidated and simplified so that patients can be seen in common locations. General medical practitioners can be supported as they implement MH/SUD treatment, including costly pharmacologic intervention, by onsite MH/SUD specialists colocated and interacting in a single clinical setting. Similarly, colocation enables MH/SUD specialists to have access to needed physical health care for their patients [10].

Most general medical health plans have not understood the value that can be derived by supporting MH/SUD services more aggressively as a part of physical health care. Many, however, are engaged in the steps immediately preceding this activity. First, they understand and agree with the premises underlying the benefits of integrated care vis-a-vis the overall improved quality of care. Second, because those most in support of integrated care are health plans specializing in Medicaid and Medicare populations and the Veterans Administration system, they have enrolled populations with great need for and potential benefit from integrated care. That is, their enrollees have a significant incidence of physical and MH/SUD issues, high and often unnecessary service use, and a high likelihood for poor clinical outcomes. In sum, all have the greatest opportunity to benefit from integrated services through altered financial approaches to service support.

EFFECT OF FUNDING CLINICAL SERVICES THROUGH PHYSICAL HEALTH BENEFITS

Perhaps the greatest concern that MH/SUD clinicians and psychiatric administrators have about funding MH/SUD services through physical health benefits is that patients who have MH/SUDs and their providers will fare poorly when competing with other medical specialties for health care funds. As noted earlier, when MH/SUD benefits are managed independently, treatment is supported for only a small minority of those with illness. Even those for whom support is provided receive less-than-optimal total health care, whether for MH/SUD needs in medicine or for physical health needs in psychiatry. In fact, since the introduction of managed behavioral health in the early 1980s, the percentage of the total health care dollar used for MH/SUDs has dropped from 6%–8% to 2%–4% (excluding costs associated with psychotropic medication, most of which are prescribed in the non-MH/SUD sector).

Because separate MH/SUD funding has fared so poorly for behavioral health, and because independently managed benefits significantly curtail clinicians' ability to provide coordinated care to patients (Table 1), the transformation of the health system to one in which assessment and treatment of MH/SUDs becomes an integral part of physical health benefits has appeal. Perhaps the most important effect of the transition will be that clinicians, regardless of the discipline in which they are trained, will take responsibility for both physical health and MH/SUD outcomes, regardless of where patients are seen.

Table 1
Administration of independent MH/SUD and physical health benefits

Patients	Same
Network providers	Separate
Member and provider support	Separate
Approval process	Separate
Care management support	Separate
Coding and billing	Separate
Claims processing	Separate
Data warehousing and actuarial analysis	Separate
Payment pool	Separate
Interaction of systems	None

Practitioners from both general medical and MH/SUD disciplines, however, will be asked to align all health outcomes in the context of a system designed to facilitate the interaction of physical health and MH/SUD professionals and services and to assure mutual support.

No longer will it be necessary to "discharge" a patient from an inpatient general or specialty medical service and then "readmit" the patient to a psychiatric service. As in the rest of medicine, patients will be "transferred" to the clinical location with the greatest safety and potential therapeutic value to the patient, without administrative hassle. Reimbursement considerations will be no greater than if a patient were transferred from surgery to medicine. No longer will the clinicians caring for patients be members of independent provider networks, requiring a "cold call" to an "800" number to find out if there is a clinician available to assist a patient. MH/SUD clinicians will be members of the same networks as other doctors, as identifiable and accessible as other clinicians serving a population.

Reimbursement procedures will encourage MH/SUD clinicians to practice and be available to patients where the majority are seen, that is, in the primary care setting. Further, impediments to medical care for patients who have MH/SUDs will be reduced, because more patients who have MH/SUDs will be seen in the physical health setting. Even patients who have severe and persistent MH/SUDs and who continue to be seen in the psychiatric setting will have better access to physical health services, because an integrated payment process does not penalize general medical practitioners from working in the MH/SUD setting, nor does it discriminate against patients who have MH/SUD by restricting payment for medical tests ordered and performed in mental health settings.

The stigma of having a MH/SUD should also become less of an issue. In the present environment, treatment for erectile dysfunction and genital herpes are the subjects of national television advertisements. Depression and anxiety are no more sensitive but are stigmatized as much by their separation from the rest of medicine as by the nature of the illnesses themselves. Making care for MH/SUDs a part of physical health care could do more to destigmatize mental health problems than any attempts through national MH/SUD awareness campaigns.

Despite the apparent value introduced by making MH/SUD benefits a part of physical health benefits, most payers still reimburse for MH/SUD services and service providers from funding pools separate from those for physical health. As a result, few general medical hospitals and clinics are interested in introducing MH/SUD services for their patients. Billing for such services is complicated, and levels of reimbursement are miniscule in comparison with most other medical specialties. Why would hospital and clinic administrators wish to invest in clinical programs that predictably will lose money when compared others services they could develop?

There also is little incentive for MH/SUD clinical services to address their patients' physical health problems. Although professional fees for physical health practitioners are paid on par with services delivered in other clinical locations, the tests that they order, the procedures that they perform, and the consultations that they request in the mental health setting are not reimbursed through separate MH/SUD funding pools. Therefore, for patients who have MH/SUD to receive physical health attention, they must be transferred to the medical setting. Sometimes, if the patient is hospitalized on a psychiatric unit or is being seen in a stand-alone psychiatric emergency room, an ambulance must be called to transport the patient to a general medical facility, at great expense and inconvenience.

The opportunities for improved quality of care for patients who have MH/SUDs seen in the general medical setting and for patients who have MH/SUD and concurrent physical health problems abound if MH/SUD benefits became a part of physical health benefits. Integrated outpatient MH/SUD and physical health services, which have been shown in a variety of clinical settings to lead to improved clinical outcomes and to lower total health care costs [12–17], are possible because primary care physicians and their MH/SUD colleagues can work in the same setting to care for patients presenting with either independent or concurrent illness.

If MH/SUD services were supported through physical health benefits, it also would be possible to create financially sustainable inpatient integrated treatment programs (ie, medical psychiatry units). Payment for specialty medical tests and procedures would become standard for patients who have psychotic and even less severe psychiatric illness co-occurring with heart disease, diabetes, or a new onset of cancer. Personnel could be trained to address both medical and psychiatric illness aggressively in a medically and psychiatrically safe environment, because competing medical and behavioral funding pools would no longer vie to avoid the costs of hospitalization in this group of patients who have a high use of medical resources.

Just as importantly, because improved outcomes for patients would become the center of attention by health plans interested in lowering costs in patients who have MH/SUDs, rather than avoiding payment for services outside a prescribed and controlled disciplinary domain, it would be possible to support the development of collaborative MH/SUD and physical health clinical programs that would prevent high-cost presentations (eg, delirium prevention programs [18]), shorten illness episodes, prevent illness progression (eg, brief screening and intervention for alcohol abuse [19]), and identify high-risk populations and lower costs through early symptom recognition and timely intervention (eg, use of INTERMED case finding and intervention [20]), among others. Integration of general medical and psychiatric evidence-based services throughout the health system would become possible.

STEPS TO IMPROVE PSYCHIATRIC SERVICE ACCESS IN THE GENERAL MEDICAL SETTING
Outpatient Services
Many forward-looking hospitals and clinics have initiated attempts to integrate general medical and psychiatric inpatient and outpatient services despite the hostile financial environment. Primary care clinics insert mental health professionals, mainly nurses, psychologists, and social workers, into their clinic settings in an attempt to reverse the negative impact that depression and other MH/SUDs have on clinical outcomes in general medical patients. These MH/SUD specialists generally are unable to cover their salaries through billing and collection; thus it is necessary to subsidize their contributions with the earnings from clinic physicians' or facility fees. Clinics that have taken these preliminary steps will be the first to benefit from the incorporation of MH/SUD claims into physical health claims. This benefit will require the negotiated provider/medical health plan's hourly rates for MH/SUD clinical services to be sufficient to cover mental health workers' salaries.

One of the biggest drawbacks in setting up a primary care clinic for integrated physical health and MH/SUD services in the current fiscal environment is that closer attention is given to the cost of hiring the MH/SUD personnel than to their ability to improve patient symptoms. Thus, MH/SUD professional skills that are ill suited to the patients seen in a physical health care environment lead to de facto support for MH/SUD services that are segregated and devoid of focus on holistic improvement of patient outcomes. For instance, many chronically ill primary care patients have concurrent depression. If MH/SUD staff, such as a low-cost masters level "counselor," in the primary care setting merely provide supportive therapy or crisis intervention but are not sufficiently trained to provide an evidence-based form of psychotherapy, such as cognitive behavioral therapy or interpersonal psychotherapy, little value is realized by the patient or the primary care provider.

Perhaps more importantly, prescriptions for antidepressants have documented evidence of efficacy, but 70% or more are written by primary care physicians who use practices that lead to limited resolution of symptoms (ie, lower doses, inadequate trials of medications) [3,21]. In the primary care setting, psychiatrists are considered "too expensive" to hire and support a clinic's non-psychiatrist physicians, but they are the only mental health professionals who have the training and skills needed to reverse the reasons that so few primary care patients who have mental disorders improve although receiving apparently appropriate medication. Psychiatrists could help monitor important issues, such as patients' failing to fill their antidepressant prescription because of poor education about depression, inadequate doses being given, initiation of alternative medications when patients do not respond, or patients stopping medication prematurely. Primary care physicians have prescriptive ability, but it does not mean that they achieve anticipated evidence-based outcomes when antidepressants are used.

Inpatient Services

From a fiscal standpoint in today's climate, the reimbursement incentive is much greater for health care administrators to build stand-alone psychiatric facilities for inpatient care of patients who have MH/SUD. A limited number of general hospitals, however, now recognize the substantial costs incurred when patients who have physical illnesses and concurrent MH/SUDs are admitted to general medical and surgical units [5]. General hospital administrators in these facilities have documented that losses associated with extended lengths of stay and the use of one-on-one nursing observation far exceed the costs associated with development of integrated treatment units (medical psychiatry units) and support for proactive, evidence-focused, integrated psychiatric services [22]. As a result, more than 25 integrated inpatient medical psychiatry units are known to be in operation in the United States. They also are growing in popularity in other countries, including the Netherlands, Canada, Australia, and Japan.

From an economic standpoint, hospitals that have done their homework have licensed their medical psychiatry units as internal medicine beds. This approach allows the delivery of full general medical and psychiatric services, and reimbursement for ancillary services (eg, laboratory tests, radiography, and medical procedures) becomes part of standard procedure. Hospitals maximize income from inpatient care, save money on one-on-one nursing observation because of the psychiatric capabilities on the unit [23,24], benefit in the diagnostic related-group reimbursement scheme by discharging complex patients an average of 4 days sooner [25,26], and have fewer unnecessary hospital days arising from placement issues. The biggest beneficiaries with these medical psychiatry units, however, are the patients. They receive aggressive assessment and intervention for both their physical and psychiatric illness immediately and simultaneously on admission, have more rapid and robust clinical improvement, and are discharged to less restrictive outpatient locations [27].

Many patients admitted to general hospitals with concurrent medical and psychiatric illnesses may not require the special characteristics of a medical psychiatry unit. General hospitals with medical psychiatric units in operation, however, have the capability to recognize the important interaction between physical and MH/SUD services and possess augmented hospital-wide integrated psychiatric capabilities that can identify potential problems proactively before crises emerge [28–30]. These integrated programs address the needs of the large number of complex patients in the medical setting who have concurrent psychiatric illness, for whom admission or transfer to a medical psychiatry unit is not necessary or feasible. In addition to helping medical staff deal with the psychologic, social, and health system issues these patients face, they are equipped to add preventive services, such as delirium prevention programs [18,31,32], that reduce mortality, morbidity, and cost.

DISCUSSION

This article discusses the barriers created by the current health care reimbursement system, in which MH/SUD service support is segregated from that of physical health, whether carved-out through independently managed behavioral health organizations or carved-in but with retention of separate general medical and behavioral business practices. It then provides data showing that altering the system to make MH/SUDs a part of physical health benefits would lead to a greater number of patients who have MH/SUDs being treated, to more effective treatment of complex patients who have concurrent physical health and MH/SUDs in the medical and psychiatric settings, to better coordination of cross-disciplinary clinical care, and to lower total health care costs. Finally, it describes inpatient and outpatient programs that have developed integrated services despite a reimbursement system that makes it difficult to do so and remain economically viable.

Because most psychiatric administrators must run their clinical programs and make a profit, or at least break even, and because MH/SUD providers need to make a living wage, many will question the purpose of this article. At present, physical health and MH/SUD services are paid from separate funding. What, in today's health care environment, can be done to alter this situation, and are the advantages worth the effort?

It remains difficult for integrated outpatient programs in primary care to succeed, particularly when the focus is on the cost of MH/SUD personnel in the physical health setting rather than on patient outcomes. Nonetheless, some general medical and behavioral health plans are increasingly willing to create specialized payment procedures because they recognize the impact of MH/SUDs on physical health outcomes and cost and the positive benefits of integrated services. Further, customers of these same health plans are beginning to demand integrated services for the constituents for whom they are purchasing health insurance. Employers and government programs now recognize that untreated MH/SUDs in primary care leads to higher total health care and disability costs and greater total public program costs (ie, the composite of health, education, social services, and correctional costs). They want MH/SUDs to be treated as effectively as enrollees' physical health problems and in coordination with them.

These trends provide opportunities to negotiate contracts for solvent integrated programs, if general medical and MH/SUD administrators are willing to work together in presenting descriptions of coordinated services to general medical health plans. Because they already are paying the price for ineffectively treated, complex, fragile, expensive patients whose benefit costs shift from the behavioral to the general medical pool [5], many are willing to consider reimbursement adjustments that will support MH/SUD teams in primary care adequately. Until MH/SUD benefits become a part of physical health benefits, which will take several years to accomplish, this approach to improve local reimbursement should not be overlooked.

Internal medicine units in general hospitals typically run at capacity. Few open beds are available, and most internal medicine departments would prefer to avoid attracting patients who have comorbid psychiatric illness. Most internal medicine departments, therefore, are reluctant to consider the development of medical psychiatry units using space designated for their patients.

What the administrators of these units fail to realize is that more than a quarter of their admissions have concurrent MH/SUDs that interfere with treatment of the patient's physical illness, lead to the need for constant observation, and/or extend the patient's length of stay [33]. Two percent to 4% of these patients would receive substantially better clinical care if treated in a medical psychiatry unit. Such an outcome-changing service will never become available unless the administrators of the medical units are willing to collaborate with psychiatry in developing a unit that meets the licensure requirements for medical beds. With medical bed designation, the integrated unit will be able to treat safely all levels of medical acuity addressed on other general medical units; ensure coordination of cross-disciplinary assessment and treatment; and reduce high-cost service needs, such as constant observation, while shortening length of stay.

Even in today's health care environment, medical psychiatry units, as formulated in this article, make a profit for general hospitals, reduce total cost of care, and discharge patients who are healthier and thus less likely to need posthospitalization service and readmission. General medical hospitals willing to consider innovative approaches to some of their most complex patients have substantial opportunity in the inpatient area despite a presently segregated reimbursement system.

Up to this point, this article has discussed short-term opportunities to influence complex, comorbid patient outcomes. Local or regional negotiations make it possible to set up special payment scenarios that bring value to patients and to the health system. Ultimately, however, system-wide implementation of integrated care practices will be necessary to reverse negative outcomes associated with comorbid medical and psychiatric illness. For psychiatry to influence such progress, psychiatric administrators must understand that it is better for them to be at the general medical negotiating table than to attempt to negotiate favorable terms on their own, largely from the scraps that are left after physical health service negotiations have reached completion.

Psychiatry clearly will need to argue its case and compete with other medical specialty demands; however, it is in a particularly good position to do so in the current health care environment. If nothing else, the separation of general medical and psychiatric benefits has served to document the importance of psychiatric care. Illness in no other discipline is as prevalent as or has more impact on outcomes than psychiatric illness in the general medical setting. Further, this situation can change only with effective treatment, supported through the coordination of medical and psychiatric services. Likewise, if psychiatrists are not able to represent patient interests in the face of data that indicate so overwhelmingly that evidence-based psychiatric services need to be available in every medical setting and that physical health services need to be bolstered in the psychiatric setting, psychiatry does not deserve the additional funding such a transition could bring.

By partnering with their medical colleagues during annual provider contract negotiations, psychiatric administrators and mental health practitioners who recognize this opportunity can initiate processes of change through which behavioral health benefits can become a part of physical health benefits. Among other proposals in negotiating a new way to support MH/SUD care are that

1. MH/SUD clinicians will be within physical health networks
2. Credentialing will be a single-standard process for both physical and MH/SUD clinicians
3. All future insurance contracts with general medical health plans will include MH/SUD treatment as a part of basic health benefits (one payment pool)
4. Claims adjudication processes (coding, billing, payment) will be common for physical and MH/SUD
5. Approval processes (medical necessity, copayment/coinsurance, annual and lifetime limits, and others) will be equivalent for general medical and MH/SUD
6. Quality-improvement programs will be integrated

References

[1] Narrow WE, Rae DS, Robins LN, et al. Revised prevalence estimates of mental disorders in the United States: using a clinical significance criterion to reconcile 2 surveys' estimates. Arch Gen Psychiatry 2002;59(2):115–23.

[2] Kessler RC, Demler O, Frank RG, et al. Prevalence and treatment of mental disorders, 1990 to 2003. N Engl J Med 2005;352(24):2515–23.

[3] Wang PS, Demler O, Kessler RC. Adequacy of treatment for serious mental illness in the United States. Am J Public Health 2002;92(1):92–8.

[4] Wang PS, Lane M, Olfson M, et al. Twelve-month use of mental health services in the United States: results from the National Comorbidity Survey Replication. Arch Gen Psychiatry 2005;62(6):629–40.

[5] Kathol R, Saravay S, Lobo A, et al. Epidemiologic trends and costs of fragmentation. Med Clin North Am 2006;90:549–72.

[6] Kathol RG, McAlpine D, Kishi Y, et al. General medical and pharmacy claims expenditures in users of behavioral health services. J Gen Intern Med 2005;20(2):160–7.

[7] Druss BG, von Esenwein SA. Improving general medical care for persons with mental and addictive disorders: systematic review. Gen Hosp Psychiatry 2006;28(2):145–53.

[8] Miller BJ, Paschall CB 3rd, Svendsen DP. Mortality and medical comorbidity among patients with serious mental illness. Psychiatr Serv 2006;57(10):1482–7.

[9] HayGroup. Health care plan design and cost trends. 1988 through 1998. Available at: http://www.naphs.org/News/hay99/hay99.html. Accessed December 26, 2007.

[10] Kathol R, Gatteau S. Healing body and mind: a critical issue for health care reform. Westport (CN): Praeger; 2007.

[11] Rosenheck RA, Druss B, Stolar M, et al. Effect of declining mental health service use on employees of a large corporation. Health Aff (Millwood) 1999;18(5):193–203.

[12] Anton RF, O'Malley SS, Ciraulo DA, et al. Combined pharmacotherapies and behavioral interventions for alcohol dependence: the COMBINE study: a randomized controlled trial. JAMA 2006;295(17):2003–17.

[13] Katon W, Russo J, Sherbourne C, et al. Incremental cost-effectiveness of a collaborative care intervention for panic disorder. Psychol Med 2006;36(3):353–63.

[14] Katon W, Unutzer J, Fan MY, et al. Cost-effectiveness and net benefit of enhanced treatment of depression for older adults with diabetes and depression. Diabetes Care 2006;29(2): 265–70.

[15] Fink P, Rosendal M, Toft T. Assessment and treatment of functional disorders in general practice: the extended reattribution and management model–an advanced educational program for nonpsychiatric doctors. Psychosomatics 2002;43(2):93–131.

[16] Toft T. Managing patients with functional somatic symptoms in general practice. Aarhus (Denmark): Departments of General Practice and Psychiatry, University of Aarhus; 2004.

[17] Parthasarathy S, Mertens J, Moore C, et al. Utilization and cost impact of integrating substance abuse treatment and primary care. Med Care 2003;41(3):357–67.

[18] Inouye SK, Bogardus ST Jr, Williams CS, et al. The role of adherence on the effectiveness of nonpharmacologic interventions: evidence from the delirium prevention trial. Arch Intern Med 2003;163(8):958–64.

[19] Kaner EF, Beyer F, Dickinson HO, et al. Effectiveness of brief alcohol interventions in primary care populations. Cochrane Database Syst Rev 2007;(2):CD004148.

[20] de Jonge P, Latour CH, Huyse FJ. Implementing psychiatric interventions on a medical ward: effects on patients' quality of life and length of hospital stay. Psychosom Med 2003;65(6): 997–1002.

[21] Wang PS, Berglund P, Olfson M, et al. Failure and delay in initial treatment contact after first onset of mental disorders in the National Comorbidity Survey Replication. Arch Gen Psychiatry 2005;62(6):603–13.

[22] Kathol RG, Harsch HH, Hall RC, et al. Categorization of types of medical/psychiatry units based on level of acuity. Psychosomatics 1992;33(4):376–86.

[23] Blumenfield M, Milazzo J, Orlowski B. Constant observation in the general hospital. Psychosomatics 2000;41(4):289–93.

[24] Worley LL, Kunkel EJ, Gitlin DF, et al. Constant observation practices in the general hospital setting: a national survey. Psychosomatics 2000;41(4):301–10.

[25] Sloan D, Yokley J, Gottesman H, et al. A five year study on the interactive effects of depression and physical illness on psychiatric unit length of stay. Psychosom Med 1999;61(1):21–5.

[26] Young J, Harsch H. Length of stay on a psychiatry medicine unit. Gen Hosp Psychiatry 1989;11(1):31–5.

[27] Kishi Y, Kathol RG. Integrating medical and psychiatric treatment in an inpatient medical setting. The type IV program. Psychosomatics 1999;40(4):345–55.

[28] Huyse F, Stiefel F, Jonge Pd. Identifiers, or "red flags," of complexity or need for integrated care. Med Clin North Am 2006;90:703–12.

[29] Huyse FJ. From consultation to complexity of care prediction and health service needs assessment. J Psychosom Res 1997;43(3):233–40.

[30] Stiefel F, Huyse F, Söllner W, et al. Operationalizing integrated care on a clinical level: the INTERMED project. Med Clin North Am 2006;90:713–58.

[31] Marcantonio ER, Flacker JM, Wright RJ, et al. Reducing delirium after hip fracture: a randomized trial. J Am Geriatr Soc 2001;49(5):516–22.

[32] Tabet N, Hudson S, Sweeney V, et al. An educational intervention can prevent delirium on acute medical wards. Age Ageing 2005;34(2):152–6.

[33] Kathol R, Stoudemire A, JR WMR. Strategic integration of inpatient and outpatient medical-psychiatry services. In: The textbook of consultation-liaison psychiatry. 2nd edition. Washington, DC: APPI Press; 2002. p. 995–1014.

Psychiatr Clin N Am 31 (2008) 27–42

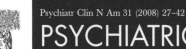

PSYCHIATRIC CLINICS
OF NORTH AMERICA

Whither Hospital and Academic Psychiatry?

George E. Tesar, MD

Department of Psychiatry & Psychology, Cleveland Clinic Neurological Institute, Cleveland Clinic
Foundation, 9500 Euclid Avenue, Desk P57, Cleveland, OH 44195, USA

No margin - no mission.
- Anonymous CEO

F or better or worse, health care delivery in the United States is a business. Like any business, if it spends more than it earns, it cannot survive. If it cannot survive, then obviously it cannot pursue the mission—no matter how worthy or essential—it set out to fulfill.

Since the mid- to late 1970s, the business of American medicine has been under mounting pressure to control its expenses [1–3]. Following World War II, a massive infusion of largely government-funded grants supported unrestrained growth of American medical services and research. In the lap of government-funded luxury and plentiful National Institutes of Health (NIH) research grants, academic medical centers evolved in scope and complexity to become powerful and influential institutions [3]. Eventually, however, skyrocketing costs led to recognition by the mid-1970s of a "crisis in American health care" [1].

In response, the government initiated cost-cutting measures that heralded a painful transition from a nearly 40-year era of health care expansion. Ending in the mid-1980s, the era nostalgically named the "Golden Age of Medicine" collided with the era of managed care. With a business-minded focus on the bottom line, for-profit management companies emerged in the mid- to late 1980s with the simple, straightforward goal of reducing cost. Intensive management led initially to sharp decreases in health care expenditures, but the almost exclusive emphasis on cost coupled with heavy-handed intrusions on physician authority and the doctor–patient relationship caused wide-spread dissatisfaction among health care professionals and the patients they served [3].

Among the medical subspecialties, psychiatry was the first and hardest hit by managed care [4,5]. Employing a time-intensive, cognitive practice model short

E-mail address: tesarg@ccf.org

0193-953X/08/$ – see front matter
doi:10.1016/j.psc.2007.11.005

on revenue-generating technology, psychiatry was especially vulnerable. Apart from nonclinical revenues generated by research, contractual, and educational grants, many academic psychiatry departments relied heavily on inpatient revenues to cover their expenses [2]. Long hospital stays were desirable because they fattened departmental coffers. Management techniques that sharply reduced length of stay, therefore, threatened the viability of important departmental endeavors, particularly the non–revenue-generating activities devoted to education and training. The impact of discounted professional fees and an escalating demand for clinical service compounded the problem by reducing time and resources available for psychiatry's academic mission.

So that it not wither on the vine of academic medicine, psychiatry, like other branches of medicine, must develop new and innovative ways to pursue its tripartite mission of healing, teaching, and investigation. It could be said that an answer to the question, "Whither do we go?" was articulated early in the twentieth century by Adolf Meyer, "father of American psychiatry." He and his followers called upon the "alienists" to broaden their base beyond the asylum and reintegrate with the rest of medicine [6]. The essence of his holistic vision had been hinted at by Benjamin Rush more than 100 years earlier, and by others before him. Unfortunately, and for a variety of reasons, American medicine still has been unable to incorporate fully Rush's simple notion that "Man is said to be a compound of soul and body ... so intimately united ... that one cannot be moved without the other" [7].

American medicine, and psychiatry in particular, continues to face the challenge and the opportunity to realize this long-held vision fully. Arguably, psychiatry's survival depends on its ability to maintain strong relationships with its colleagues and other partners in the medical community. The strength of that partnership will depend on the value psychiatry's membership brings to the health care team, a value measured by (1) the accessibility of mental health care services; (2) the quality of mental health care provided; (3) the effectiveness of interdisciplinary communication; and (4) a favorable impact on the cost of health care in general.

If psychiatrists are to bring value to the health care team, training a renewable force of such psychiatrists is essential. Have psychiatrists been trained to bring maximal value to the health care team? Is such training being provided now? Given the current health care climate, will sufficient funding be available to train this renewable force optimally? This article addresses these questions from an historical-developmental perspective, identifies current challenges, and outlines opportunities for further growth and development.

THE ORIGINS AND DEVELOPMENT OF THE TEACHING HOSPITAL

> Competent practitioners of medicine can be trained in but one way, and that is in the hospital and in the dispensary, which are the clinical laboratories in which the students must study.

Arthur Dean Bevan, Chairman of the Council on Medical Education of the American Medical Association, Meeting of 11 June 1924, Agenda and Minutes of the Business Meetings of the Council on Medical Education and Hospitals [8].

Following the Civil War, the American medical school, until then often a free-standing entity, evolved to its current status as a cornerstone of most universities. The advances in medical education signaled by Flexner's groundbreaking report on medical education [9] necessitated a clinical training experience that supplemented the scientific training of the first 2 years. Hospitals, which had opposed mixing the needs of medical students and patients, began to accommodate the needs of medical schools, especially as the quality of their students improved. In the forefront of this evolution in medical education, Johns Hopkins Medical School, which opened in 1893, was the first to provide hospital-based training in a large, well-equipped hospital for its students and graduates [8]. As the twentieth century unfolded, Johns Hopkins set the standard for hospital-based medical education in a university setting.

The idea of teaching medicine in hospitals, previously eschewed by the public, assumed a new importance. After World War I, advances in technology, a national mandate to incorporate research into patient care, and a growing supply of medical students and graduates were among the factors responsible for the growth of teaching hospitals. Although even then it was recognized that the hospitalized patient was not representative of what most physicians would encounter during their careers, the hospital setting provided a convenient, ready, and stable supply of patients to satisfy the requirements of medical training. In 1923, Francis W. Peabody, professor at Harvard Medical School, an influential educator and a strong advocate of the teaching hospital concept, wrote: "There are few influences that exert as elevating an effect on the standard of professional work in a hospital as the presence in it of medical teaching. This is so true that the phrase 'teaching hospital' is almost synonymous with a good hospital" [10].

The growth of teaching hospitals coincided with a national mandate for a more scientific approach to medical care. Advances in medical care such as salvorsan for treatment of syphilis (1910), insulin for diabetes (1922), and liver extract for pernicious anemia (1926) provided compelling evidence of the important role scientific research and a scientific understanding of the body had for the medical profession. These developments corresponded with the strategic plan of the Rockefeller Foundation, which in 1929 made an explicit decision to invest in medical science [11].

PSYCHIATRY IN THE TEACHING HOSPITAL

Not only was the Rockefeller Foundation interested in advancing the physical health of mankind through medical science; it also had an abiding interest in advancing social stability [11]. Alan Gregg, the Rockefeller Foundation program director for medical sciences, explained its interest in noting that physicians increasingly "are being looked to for knowledge that will help in interpreting as well as in guiding the behavior of man." Because "medicine lacks sufficient basic data in these fields to meet such a demand," what was needed was the knowledge of the "ideal psychiatrist" that might speak to these kinds of "economic, moral, social and spiritual losses" [11].

Gregg found that "ideal psychiatrist" in Adolf Meyer, a Swiss-born neuropathologist who introduced the European term, "psychiatry," to America and also the important synthetic concept, psychobiology [11]. As espoused by Meyer, psychobiology was a monistic philosophy that considered psyche and soma as separate dimensions of the same thing [6]. In contrast to the Kraepelinian conceptualization of mental disorder as an organic defect, Meyer offered an approach that focused on personality as a functional outcome of the interaction between environment and individual biology. For Meyer, mental disturbance, rather than reflecting a structural defect of either mind or body, represented a maladjustment or maladaptation to an individual's environment. Meyer viewed maladjustment not just as result but also as a cause of societal disturbance. The physician's responsibility, therefore, extended beyond the individual to society as a whole. From Meyer's point of view, the physician had the dual role of maintaining societal as well as personal fitness. The ideal physician to accomplish this task, Meyer proposed, was to be called a "psychiatrist."

To Gregg, psychobiology and the new profession of psychiatry were precisely what the Rockefeller Foundation was interested in funding. Unfortunately, Meyer's psychobiology lacked a credible scientific foundation. This lack forced Gregg, in his campaign to convince Rockefeller Foundation trustees of its merit, to promote a refurbished, innovative version of psychobiology that he himself dubbed "psychosomatic medicine" [9]. Psychosomatic medicine was presented as a branch of medical science that used laboratory methods to study the impact of the psyche and of behavior and societal influences on health.

The Rockefeller Foundation extended support for research in psychosomatic medicine to its clinical application in general hospitals. A notable fund recipient and representative of the Meyerian push toward integration of psychiatry and medicine was Edward G. Billings, Director of the Psychiatric Liaison Department, a division of the Department of Psychiatry at the Colorado University School of Medicine. With a primary goal of furthering the concept, Billings described his department and its many services in the August 19, 1936 issue of the *Journal of the American Medical Association* [12]. He described the "three broad aims" around which the department was organized:

1. To sensitize the physicians and students to the opportunities offered them by every patient, no matter what complaint or ailment is present, for the use of a "common sense" psychiatric approach for the betterment of the patient's condition, and for making the patient better fitted to handle his problems— somatic or personality-determined or both.
2. To establish psychobiology as an integral working part of the professional thinking of physicians and students of all branches of medicine.
3. To instil [sic] in the physicians and students the need the patient-public has for a more tangible and practical conception in the sense of "prevention" of

mental and personality disorders, per se, but rather in the sense of prevention of false thinking, misconception, misunderstanding, folklore and tabus
[sic], which make it difficult for the patient to accept help or to allow the physician to be of help.

Billings emphasized the important role of the liaison psychiatrist as teacher of
students, residents, and non-psychiatric physicians. In addition to formal lectures, ward rounds with the students and then with the medical team were
used as occasions to teach the principles of psychiatric assessment and treatment. When communicating either verbally or in writing, he stressed the
importance of using language that presented "a clear and concise verbal picture" of the patient's complaint and to "avoid nosologic psychiatric diagnosis
in favor of a summarizing sentence or two that neutralizes any antipathy
that might exist for 'big words'." In the spirit of Meyerian psychobiology
and the community psychiatry movement of 30 years later, Billings called
for amplification of the focus beyond the walls of the general hospital to the
community at large in which it existed:

> A constant effort is made to sensitize the student and hospital physician to the
> sociological needs of the community, as to how patients' symptoms are reper-
> cussions of general economic problems, as to his responsibility to his commu-
> nity and patient, and as to how he can use the available resources [12].

Others followed the example set by Billings. Funded by Rockefeller Foundation seed monies, similar services open at Harvard's Massachusetts General
Hospital under the direction of Stanley Cobb [13], the Institute of Pennsylvania
Hospital, the Chicago Institute of Psychoanalysis directed by Franz Alexander,
Yale University's Institute of Human Relations headed by John F. Fulton [11],
and Washington University in St. Louis led by Carlyle Jacobsen [14]. Fulton's
and Jacobsen's work in the Yerkes Primate Laboratory at Yale University led
to early support of Freeman and Watt's work on frontal lobotomy [11,15] and
later to Paul McLean's elaboration of Papez's groundbreaking work on the
neurocircuitry of emotion that McLean dubbed "the visceral brain" and later
"the limbic system" [16].

THE ACADEMIC MEDICAL CENTER COMES OF AGE

After World War II, the union of teaching hospital and medical school enjoyed
unprecedented growth. A new term, "academic medical center," became a more
fitting descriptor of the two separate institutions that together consolidated their
strength with the aid of massive government funding for research, medical
education, and hospital growth [8]. Like the rest of medicine, psychiatry reaped
dividends from the World War II experience and thrived on the government-
funded research and program development that followed. Conscription efforts
during the war had identified a large population of men who were unfit for military duty because of mental disturbance. Following the war, there was a tremen-
dous demand for mental health services to help deal with the psychiatric

aftermath of battle exposure. In 1946, passage of the National Mental Health Act made money available for research and education and led to establishment of the National Institutes of Mental Health (NIMH) [1].

Given the teaching hospital's centrality to the mission of training doctors and the provision of health care to the American public, investing in hospital growth and development seemed essential. Passage of the Hill-Burton Act in 1947 ushered in a period of unprecedented hospital construction. General hospital psychiatric units grew to 1358 by 1984 and to 1707 by 1990 [17]. Rapid expansion of the commercial indemnity insurance industry after 1945 and enactment of Medicare and Medicaid in 1966 made health care more accessible and ensured that hospital beds were occupied. During this period of growth there was a corresponding increase in the number of medical schools and their graduates. From 1960 to 1980 the number of medical schools increased from 86 to 126, and the number of their graduates more than doubled from 6994 to 15,985 [8].

Continued expansion of medical services, however, was costly. By 1970, the rate of growth in health care expenditures had risen from 3.2% annually in the 7 years before Medicare and Medicaid legislation to 7.9% annually in the subsequent 5 years; during the same period, the corresponding inflation rate for all other services in the consumer price index had increased from 2% to 5.8% [1]. Whereas total health care expenditures in the United States were $74.9 billion in 1970, they had jumped to $253.9 billion by 1980, an increase from 7.2% to 9.1% of the gross domestic product [18].

Congress responded with legislation meant to limit spending on both hospital services and physician fees. In 1982 legislation was enacted to regulate Medicare spending by paying for episodes of care rather than the cost of delivering that care. The new prospective payment system (PPS) based reimbursement for hospital-level care on the diagnostic-related group (DRG), a predetermined measure of resource use [2,3]. The rationale behind PPS was to create incentives for efficiency by paying according to the diagnosed condition rather than on a cost-plus basis. In 1992 further legislation was introduced to limit coverage of physician fees using the Resource Based Relative Value Scale. The Balanced Budget Act of 1997, designed to balance the federal budget by 2002, had as one of its strategies reduction of Medicare payments for both hospital services and indirect medical education payments that support graduate medical education (GME). Although the impact of these and other cost-cutting tactics might be reflected in reduced spending from 1993 to 2004, their inherent limitations are evident, because by 2005 the percentage of health care expenditure per gross domestic product had risen to 16% [18].

Implementation of strategies to limit health care spending is expected to continue into the foreseeable future. Although a compelling argument can be made for redirecting attention from cost cutting to competition-based improvements in the value of health care [3], the impact of government regulation looms large until the health care community is able to provide measurable and compelling evidence of its value to the public. In the meantime preventing cost escalation without significantly compromising medicine's academic mission will be a significant challenge.

Nowhere in medicine is the challenge to demonstrate value greater than in psychiatry. Although other disciplines share this challenge, the stakes are higher in psychiatry because of its comparatively narrow revenue base, because of the enduring stigma associated with psychiatric illness and its treatment, and because identification of meaningful and measurable outcomes is perhaps more difficult for psychiatry than other medical disciplines.

FUNDING OF GRADUATE MEDICAL EDUCATION

The funds allocated for GME are intended to pay for the portion of medical training that prepares a trainee to acquire credentials necessary to practice medicine in one or more subspecialties, including primary care. The costs of training are multiple and include the salary and benefits of the trainee (resident or fellow), the stipends of faculty involved in either teaching and supervision or program administration, and other overhead costs of providing health care in an academic health center. The total cost depends on the total number of residents and fellows in training, which in turn depends (or, some would argue, should depend) on physician supply and demand [19–21].

Who pays for these costs? How is physician supply and demand regulated? The first formal, policy-minded attention to these questions occurred when Medicare was introduced in 1966 [19]. Until that time, the topic received little attention.

For 20 years following World War II, GME was supported by generous NIH research grants [1,22]. As research dollars became less plentiful, academic departments turned to clinical revenues to subsidize their academic mission. With the growth of the hospital infrastructure in the United States and the availability of third-party insurance benefits, health care use increased, as did the revenues it generated. From 1965 to 1980, academic medical centers enjoyed a 15-fold increase in income derived from patient care [22].

The enactment of PPS under Medicare in 1983 signaled an end to department-building and cost-based reimbursement and forced academic medical departments to pay closer attention to GME funding. During the legislative action that led to introduction of Medicare and Medicaid in 1966, policymakers debated the merits of using health care dollars to fund GME [19]. Although there was general agreement that dollars designated for patient care should not be used to fund medical education, it also was acknowledged that there was no permanent source of funding for GME and that educational activities enhanced patient care. Although academic departments had thrived on generous cost-based reimbursement for patient care, there was little incentive to focus attention on GME funding until the introduction of PPS. The comparatively high cost of providing care in the teaching hospital and the inability of DRG methodology to serve as a reliable measure of acuity led to enactment of explicit Medicare funding for GME.

Despite ongoing controversy over this funding mechanism, Medicare remains the largest single source of explicit GME funding [19]. Other funding sources include other federal government sources (the Department of Veterans Affairs, Medicaid, the Public Health Service, the Department of Defense, and the National Institutes of Health), state government sources (Medicaid and state programs), and the private sector (department practice plans, industry grants and contracts, department-sponsored, nonclinical revenue-generating activities [CME programs], and philanthropy) [19,21].

Medicare dollars are used to subsidize so-called "direct" and "indirect" educational costs [19,21]. The direct payments are used to cover the costs of resident salaries and benefits, department faculty compensation for teaching and supervision, and overhead costs attributable to teaching activities. Calculation of direct costs is based on the number of residents at the hospital multiplied by the hospital-specific, per-resident amount. The indirect payments are intended to cover the comparatively higher costs of providing care in a teaching hospital and are based on teaching intensity, that is, the resident-to-bed ratio. Factors that contribute to the higher cost of delivering care in a teaching hospital include charity care, specialized care, complex or high-acuity medical conditions, and research [19]. In fact, academic health centers that receive Medicare GME funding have a longer median length of stay than the average at all hospitals and bear a disproportionate share of the cost burden for charity care (43 times higher than the national average for hospitals) [20].

Proponents of Medicare GME funding, especially the indirect medical education portion, argue that these funds support the "multiple missions" of the medical schools and teaching hospitals [20]. Critics of the current Medicare funding scheme levy the following complaints [19,20]:

1. The hospital-specific per-resident amounts vary widely.
2. They are based on historical cost patterns set in 1984.
3. Payments flow to individuals responsible for managing the hospital rather than those responsible for GME.
4. Payment to teaching hospitals for GME impedes the development of residency programs in nonhospital ambulatory and managed care settings.
5. The linkage to physician workforce objectives is too weak to achieve them.
6. The linkage to Medicare services means that teaching hospitals with low Medicare use (eg, pediatric hospitals) receive little of no federal support for educational activities.

Moreover, no methodology exists to account for the hidden, indirect costs, thereby making indirect medical education funding more vulnerable to indiscriminate cuts in the effort to curb Medicare spending. As described by Koenig and colleagues [20], "the current system by which these missions are financed is a mélange of implicit and explicit subsidies, none of which is based on a clear notion of what is being paid for."

IMPACT OF THE HEALTH CARE ECONOMY ON GRADUATE MEDICAL EDUCATION IN PSYCHIATRY

Continued funding of GME under Medicare is threatened because of its uncertain management and because its cost has increased annually since Medicare was first enacted in 1984. The Balanced Budget Act of 1997, with an overarching goal of balancing the federal budget, included legislation to redress problems of cost and accountability of the current GME funding scheme. The Balanced Budget Act changed the funding of direct medical education expenses from a cost-based to a hospital-specific methodology with the intention of influencing workforce patterns by limiting the number and types of residency positions funded [19]. The Act includes limited support for GME through the period necessary for fellowship training for subspecialty board eligibility, thus restricting ability of hospitals to support fellowship training in subspecialties and thereby, it is hoped, increasing the percentage of primary care physicians [23]. The legislation also discontinues support of international medical graduates, which would have a significant impact on psychiatry, whose residency slots have been occupied increasingly by international medical graduates [23]. Subsequent iterations of the Balanced Budget Act have reduced its impact by delaying initial action and postponing the implementation of budget cuts [20].

The impact of the Balanced Budget Act has been layered onto the effects of managed care and governmental policies that have either directly or indirectly cut into resources available for GME. In response to alleged fraudulent billing for unsupervised patient care provided by residents, the Health Care Financing Administration (HCFA) imposed guidelines that link reimbursement to documented evidence of direct attending faculty involvement in resident-provided patient care [24]. Concern has been expressed that the extra time required for faculty documentation may reduce time for teaching, potentially encroach on resident autonomy, and increase the risk of reimbursement denial during concurrent review of inadequately documented but otherwise high-quality care. Similarly, the impact of managed care has forced faculty to devote more time to clinical work, which has cut into time available for teaching, supervision, and research. A recent survey of clinical teachers suggests that the impact is not critical [25]. In contrast, a study of the impact of resident teaching on radiologist productivity demonstrated that teaching reduced billed revenues by nearly 50% [26].

Managed care's impact on the viability of general hospital psychiatric services may pose an even greater potential threat to graduate education in psychiatry [17,23]. General hospitals provide the majority of inpatient psychiatric care in the United States, and they also serve as the principle site for the training of psychiatry residents, education of medical students, and performance of federally funded psychiatric research. Beginning in the 1980s general hospitals underwent a 10-year period of rapid expansion of psychiatric beds and patient days, principally because of the exemption of psychiatric service reimbursement from PPS. Escalating cost-based reimbursement prompted health insurers to enlist the help of for-profit ("carve-out") companies charged with the sole responsibility of managing the mental health portion of the patient's general health benefit. The three- to fourfold reductions in average length of stay for psychiatric inpatients and the deeply discounted per diem rates negotiated led to significant deterioration in the financial performance of general hospital psychiatric services [17,23]. Coincidentally, bed expansion plateaued after 1990 and by 2002 had dropped 30% from its peak in 1998. The number of general hospitals offering psychiatric services also dropped from 1707 in 1998 to 1285 in 2002 [27]. Similar trends in the public sector have forced general hospitals to assume the care of an increasing number of publicly funded, uninsured, and more intensely ill patients [28,29], further eroding the financial performance of general hospital psychiatric services.

Also impacting the quality of residency training in psychiatry is the seemingly ironic synergy between psychiatry and managed care in the value they both place on psychopharmacology and brief treatments. The intradisciplinary split between biologic and psychodynamic camps within psychiatry has long existed, but it intensified and grew following the 1980 publication of the third edition of the American Psychiatric Association's *Diagnostic and Statistical Manual*, DSM III [30]. Leaders in American psychiatry had argued successfully in favor of a psychiatric nosology that emphasized disorder over reaction and observable diagnostic criteria instead of assumptions about unresolved, unconscious conflict. The thrust of current psychiatry residency training has focused on learning to identify objective, verifiable, and measurable features of patient behavior, thinking, and emotion, with far less attention devoted to understanding the meaning of how patients behave, think, or feel [31]. Those who favor the latter perspective—the psychologic or psychodynamic—have lost professional standing and economic power to the psychopharmacologists and neuroscientists whose activities are directed at better understanding the pathophysiology of psychiatric disorders. This sea change in perspective appeals to the pharmaceutical industry and to the business-minded care managers who march to the mantra, "If you cannot measure it, you cannot manage it." Time and cost are easily measured but are difficult to predict when it comes to patient care, especially when the variables necessary to make accurate predictions are largely unknown. For example, one can comfortably predict that fluoxetine will impact central serotonin regulation, but predicting clinical response is subject to much greater error, especially if the psychiatrist has inadequate skill in identifying the potential psychologic, characterologic, or dynamic determinants that inform the prediction. Fortunately, as managed care has matured, its proponents have developed an appreciation of the importance of psychiatrists' being able to combine pharmacotherapy and psychotherapy skills in their assessment and treatment of patients [23].

No single generation of psychiatrists can know everything, and the training of previous generations of psychiatrists also was unbalanced by undue emphasis on the psychoanalytic perspective. The ideal will occur when it is possible to measure accurately all variables—biologic, psychologic, and social—that account for abnormal affect, cognition, and behavior. In the meantime, overemphasis on one perspective can lead to adverse outcomes. In resident training, such overemphasis risks producing a generation of psychiatrists whose knowledge of self-psychology and psychodynamic principles is so deficient that it fails to inform their practice and their instruction of subsequent generations of psychiatrists.

In the case of managed care, the well-intentioned, Meyerian-influenced, and Rockefeller Foundation–supported effort to medicalize psychiatry has unintentionally aligned itself with the time- and cost-focused interests of managed care. The emphasis on the cost effectiveness of medication management risks overvaluing pharmacotherapy [32] and relegating the role of psychiatrist to that of "pill pusher." Although this attitude may represent a cynical, narrow-minded perspective on multidisciplinary care [33], the trends in psychiatric residency training that the author has observed suggest that its dangers should not be ignored. Most psychiatrists who practice and teach in the academic health center regard "med check" as an inadequate descriptor of the breadth of care they provide. Nonetheless, non–time-based reimbursement challenges the psychiatrist to see as many "med checks" per hour as possible.

RECOMMENDATIONS FOR THE PRESENT AND FUTURE OF ACADEMIC PSYCHIATRY

This paper has focused on the teaching hospital in the academic health center, the principle site of graduate medical education in the U.S. The recommendations to be discussed pertain, therefore, to general hospital psychiatric services, and may not fully address the needs of private psychiatric hospitals, publicly-funded mental institutions, or other free-standing mental health services (eg, psychoanalytic institutes or centers). It behooves all these institutions, however, to partner with the general medical sector and thereby enhance interdisciplinary communication and access to mental healthcare services.

Advancement of psychiatry's academic mission depends on psychiatry's survival in the general hospital. Psychiatry's survival in turn depends on the value it brings to the overarching medical mission [3,34]. Unfortunately, the value of its contribution–largely dependent on inpatient revenues–has steadily diminished. General hospital psychiatry services must find ways to reverse this trend. Recommended approaches include (1) interdepartmental collaboration, (2) developing new revenue streems, (3) embracing rather than resisting change, (4) developing meaningful and measurable outcomes assessment strategies, and (5) advancing neuroscience education and research.

Interdepartmental Collaboration

Adolph Meyer recognized early-on the importance of aligning psychiatry's mission with that of the general medical establishment. Left on its own, psychiatry cannot produce the positive financial margin that keeps its mission alive. At the same time, the general hospital cannot operate effectively without psychiatric services. Efforts to do so have–in the author's experience–failed. For example, two Cleveland metropolitan area community hospitals that eliminated psychiatric inpatient units, reinstated them quickly when their general emergency services backed-up with psychiatric patients awaiting transfer elsewhere and when complaints were voiced by community representatives about the loss of accessible psychiatric services (personal communication).

Psychiatry, and the behavioral health services under its aegis (eg, health psychology, psychiatric occupational therapy, chemical dependency), must join with other disciplines (eg, oncology, preventive cardiology, epilepsy, and primary care, to name a few) in collaborative-care arrangements. Interdisciplinary teams can provide high-quality, cost-effective care by creating efficiencies and by offsetting costs related to psychiatric comorbidity (eg, greater than average length of stay due to delirium). The success of collaborative-care arrangements requires the sponsoring primary care or specialty service to share the financial burden of mental health care that is typically reimbursed at deeply discounted rates, or not at all. This might involve supporting the psychiatrist's salary or joining with psychiatry to negotiate better reimbursement rates. In return, the collaborating psychiatrist must follow through on the expectation of rapid and reliable service access, consistently high-quality care, and timely, relevant feedback. As Billings [12] and others have recommended, the feedback should be clear, concise, and free of psychiatric jargon. Unfortunately, these basic, long-established standards of psychiatric consultation are still often unmet as medical services and referring physicians continue to complain about poor access and inadequate feedback from consulting psychiatrists.

Additional Revenue Sources

These include boutique services that draw from the market of wealthy patients who can afford high-quality, high-cost services provided in a high-end environment [8]. Large departments in desirable metropolitan locations (eg, Massachusetts General Hospital) generate income from well-attended continuing medical education courses. Minnesota uses new general-tax revenues and additional appropriations from the state's tobacco settlement to finance its Medical Education and Research Cost (MERC) Trust Fund [35]. Joint ventures with for-profit businesses can be extremely lucrative, but risky as well. Relman cautioned that the "affair between teaching hospital and "the medical-industrial complex" will very likely fail, (and that) it contains the possibility of damaging academic institutions that venture too far along this path" [22]. In fact, conflict-of-interest debates have been newsworthy of late, and serve a cautionary note to those who set-out to partner with investor-owned corporations.

Embracing Change

The down-sizing of inpatient psychiatric care has forced major changes in the traditional venue and model of clinical instruction in psychiatry. The demise of the inpatient case conference and in-depth patient assessment are losses balanced perhaps by the resident's exposure to many more patients and to the multiple levels of care (eg, partial hospitalization, intensive outpatient programs) required for provision of cost-effective continuity of care. Managed care has not only forced medical subspecialties, including psychiatry, to be more cost-effective, but also more accountable for the quality of care they provide. Residents should be taught the principles of managed care so that they can responsibly incorporate the best of those principles in their future practices.

Outcomes Assessment

The importance of outcomes assessment has been long recognized and advocated [3,36], but slow to evolve. The advent of pay-for-performance (P4P) increases the pressure on all of medicine to implement strategies that identify meaningful quality outcomes and ways to measure them [3]. Although controversy surrounds P4P and medical outcomes assessment in general, and while psychiatry may face the greatest challenge among medical specialties to implement meaningful outcomes assessment, it also has the most to gain from achieving that goal. Success can enhance psychiatry's credibility, and most importantly help improve the quality of psychiatric care delivered in the general hospital. The difficulty of data acquisition and management in a paper-record environment is eased by increasing availability of the electronic medical record. The challenge is to identify meaningful data to collect, to develop strategies that assure systematic and efficient data collection at each patient-encounter, and to identify benchmarks against which to compare the data collected.

Neuroscience Education and Research

Providing more training opportunities during psychiatry residency is essential. The introduction and growth of managed behavioral health care coincided with a distinctive drop in psychiatry-led research productivity from 1987 to 2001. Whereas, the number of NIMH-funded principal investigator (PI) psychiatrists dropped from 33% to 27% of total awardees between 1987 and 2001, the percentage of PI psychologist awardees remained the same (38%), and the percentage of PI award recipients in the biologic sciences increased from 10% to 15% [37]. In 1999 and 2000, 2% of psychiatrists declared research as their primary professional activity; the corresponding figure for neurologists was 6.3% and for internal medicine subspecialties was 6.1% [37]. These and other data prompted the following comments contained in the Executive Summary of *Research Training in Psychiatry Residency: Strategies for Reform*, a publication of the Institute of Medicine [37]:

> The neural and behavioral sciences have advanced tremendously in recent years, and there has been a concomitant increase in public awareness of mental disorders. ... Unfortunately, the number of psychiatrist-researchers does not appear to be keeping pace with the unparalleled needs that currently exist in clinical brain and behavioral medicine. The need is especially acute in child and adolescent psychiatry. ... Greater financial incentives (through stipend supplements or debt repayment) and more aggressive promotion of the benefits of participation in psychiatric research are recommended as strategies to enhance trainee recruitment. ... Given that the existence of a large research effort (ie, many investigators and substantial funding) is the most salient feature of successful programs, child and adolescent psychiatry divisions and small programs in general will likely

require outside collaborations to develop a critical mass of resources for effective research training.

CONCLUSION

Until the last decade of the twentieth century, American medicine witnessed unprecedented growth. Growth of the health care infrastructure and the personnel and technology required to operate it was paid largely by the United States government and the for-profit insurance industry. Efforts to restrain health care expenditures have occurred almost continuously since the 1970s when it was first recognized that continued growth was unacceptably costly. These efforts have impacted both service delivery and training in psychiatry. The challenge psychiatrists face is to adjust their perspective on the changes they are forced to endure and view them as opportunities rather than as threats.

This core concept of crisis intervention—"in crisis there is opportunity"—was a key feature of the tiered model of preventive intervention advanced by Gerald Caplan and embraced by the community mental health movement of the 1960s and 1970s, which was supported by the President of the United States, John F. Kennedy. The President's personal enthusiasm for advances in mental health care led to passage of the 1963 National Community Mental Health Act (NCMHA). In his message to Congress, President Kennedy called for a new mental health facility that will "return mental health care to the mainstream of American medicine, and at the same time upgrade mental health services" [38]. When NCMHA funding ran out in 1975, efforts to renew it failed for the same reasons that led to tighter control of general health care spending. As a result, the vision of a comprehensive, multitiered, and well-integrated system of public mental health never materialized fully. That vision has a striking resemblance to the larger vision proposed in this article for continued integration of mental health into the larger community of health care in the United States.

References
[1] Starr P. The social transformation of American medicine. New York: Basic Books, 1982. p. 380–419.
[2] Califano JA. Radical surgery: what's next for America's health care. New York: Random House; 1994.
[3] Porter ME, Teisberg EO. Redefining healthcare: creating a value-based competition on results. Boston: Harvard Business School Press; 2006.
[4] Jellinek MS, Nurcombe B. Two wrongs don't make a right: managed care, mental health, and the marketplace. JAMA 1993;270:1737–9.
[5] Summergrad P, Herman JB, Weilburg JB, et al. Wagons ho; forward on the managed care trail. Gen Hosp Psychiatry 1995;17:251–9.
[6] Meyer A. Psychobiology: a science of man. Springfield (IL): Charles C Thomas; 1957.
[7] Rush B. Sixteen introductory lectures. Philadelphia: Bradford & Innskeep; 1811. p. 256.
[8] Ludmerer KM. Time to heal: American medical education from the turn of the century to the era of managed care. New York: Oxford University Press; 1999.
[9] Flexner A. Medical education in the United States and Canada. New York: Carnegie Foundation for the Advancement of Teaching; 1910.
[10] Peabody FW. The function of a municipal hospital. Boston Medical and Surgical Journal 1923;189:127.

[11] Pressman JD. Last resort: psychosurgery and limits of medicine. Cambridge (UK): Cambridge University Press; 1998.

[12] Billings EG. Teaching psychiatry in the medical school general hospital: a practical plan. JAMA 1936;107:635–9.

[13] Hackett TP, Cassem NH. Massachusetts General Hospital handbook of general hospital psychiatry. St. Louis: CV Mosby Company; 1978.

[14] Lipowski Z. Consultation-liaison psychiatry: the first half century. Gen Hosp Psychiatry 1986;8:305–15.

[15] Fulton JF. Frontal lobotomy and affective behavior: a neurophysiological analysis (Thomas William Salmon Lecture Series). New York: WW Norton and Company; 1951.

[16] MacLean P. Some psychiatric implications of physiological studies on frontotemporal portion of limbic system (visceral brain). Electroencephalogr Clin Neurophysiol 1952;4:407–18.

[17] Liptzin B, Gottlieb GL, Summergrad P. The future of psychiatric services in the general hospitals. Am J Psychiatry 2007;164:1468–72.

[18] Centers for Medicare & Medicaid Services, Office of the Actuary, National Health Statistics Group; U.S. Department of Commerce, Bureau of Economic Analysis, and U.S. Bureau of the Census. Table 1. National Health Expenditures Aggregate, Per Capita Amounts, Percent Distribution, and Average Annual Percent Growth, by Source of Funds: Selected Calendar Years 1960–2005. Available at: http://www.cms.hhs.gov/NationalHealthExpendData/downloads/tables.pdf. Accessed January 13, 2008.

[19] Anderson GF, Greenberg GD, Wynn BO. Graduate medical education: the policy debate. Annu Rev Public Health 2001;22:35–47.

[20] Dickinson TA. The future of financing medical education: questions about Medicare's role. Am J Med 2004;117:287–90.

[21] Jackson VP. Funding for graduate medical education. J Am Coll Radiol 2006;3:945–8.

[22] Relman AS. Who will pay for medical education in our teaching hospitals? Science 1984;226:20–3.

[23] Meyer RE, McLaughlin CJ, editors. Between mind, brain, and managed care: the now and future world of academic psychiatry. Washington, DC: American Psychiatric Press, Inc; 1998.

[24] Centers for Medicaid and Medicare Services. Documentation Guidelines for E/M Services. Available at: http://www.cms.hhs.gov/MLNEdWebGuide/25_EMDOC.asp. Accessed January 14, 2008.

[25] Woolliscroft JO, Van Harrison R, Anderson MB. Faculty views of reimbursement changes and clinical training: a survey of award-winning clinical teachers. Teach Learn Med 2002;14:77–86.

[26] Jamadar DA, Carlos R, Caoili EM, et al. Estimating the effects of informal radiology resident teaching on radiologist productivity: what is the cost of teaching? Acad Radiol 2005;12:123–8.

[27] Foley DJ, Manderscheid RW, Atay JE, et al. Highlights of organized mental health services in 2002 and major national and state trends. In: Manderscheid RW, Berry JT, editors. Mental Health, United States, 2004. Rockville (MD): US Department of Health and Human Services, publication number (SMA)-06-4195; 2006. p. 200–36.

[28] Mechanic D, McAlpine D, Olfson M. Changing patterns of psychiatric inpatient care in the United States, 1988–1994. Arch Gen Psychiatry 1998;55:785–91.

[29] Watanabe-Galloway S, Zhang W. Analysis of U.S. trends in discharges from general hospitals for episodes of serious mental illness, 1995–2002. Psychiatr Serv 2007;58:496–506.

[30] American Psychiatric Association. Diagnostic and statistical manual of mental disorders. 3rd edition. Washington, DC: American Psychiatric Association; 1980.

[31] Luhrmann TM. Of 2 minds: the growing disorder in american psychiatry. New York: Alfred A. Knopf; 2000.

[32] Goldsmith RJ, Paris M, Riba MB. Negative aspects of collaborative treatment. In: Riba MB, Balon R, editors. Psychopharmacology and psychotherapy: a collaborative approach. Washington, DC: American Psychiatric Press, Inc; 1999. p. 33–64.

[33] Balon R. Positive aspects of collaborative care. In: Riba MB, Balon R, editors. Psychophar-macology and psychotherapy: a collaborative approach. Washington, DC: American Psychiatric Press, Inc; 1999. p. 1–32.

[34] Pincus HA, Page AEK, Druss B, et al. Can psychiatry cross the quality chasm? Improving the quality of health care for mental and substance use conditions. Am J Psychiatry 2007;164: 712–9.

[35] Blewett LA, Weslowski V. New roles for states in financing graduate medical education: Minnesota's trust fund: how one state is using tobacco-settlement funds to bolster training of health professionals. Health Aff 2000;19:248–52.

[36] Outcomes assessment in clinical practice. In: Sederer LI, Dickey B, editors. Baltimore (MD): Williams & Wilkins; 1996.

[37] Institute of Medicine. Research training in psychiatry residency: strategies for reform. Washington, DC: The National Academies Press; 2003.

[38] Borus JF. Community psychiatry. In: Nicholi AM, editor. The new Harvard guide to psychiatry. Cambridge (MA): The Belknap Press of Harvard University Press; 1988. p. 780–96.

Applying the Institute of Medicine Quality Chasm Framework to Improving Health Care for Mental and Substance Use Conditions

Donna J. Keyser, PhD, MBA[a],*, Jeanie Knox Houtsinger, BA[b,c], Katherine Watkins, MD, MSHS[d], Harold Alan Pincus, MD[a,c,e]

[a]RAND-University of Pittsburgh Health Institute, 4570 Fifth Avenue, Suite 600, Pittsburgh, PA 15213, USA
[b]Department of Psychiatry, Western Psychiatric Institute and Clinic, 3811 O'Hara Street, Suite E279, Pittsburgh, PA 15213, USA
[c]Robert Wood Johnson Foundation National Program Depression in Primary Care: Linking Clinical and System Strategies, University of Pittsburgh Medical Center, 160 North Craig Street, Suite 222, Pittsburgh, PA 15213, USA
[d]RAND Corporation, 1776 Main Street, PO Box 2138, Santa Monica, CA 90407, USA
[e]Department of Psychiatry, Columbia University, New York-Presbyterian Hospital, 1051 Riverside Drive, Unit 09, New York, NY 10032, USA

With the release of its seminal report, *To Err Is Human: Building a Safer Health System* (2000), the Institute of Medicine (IOM) launched a nationwide call for action to improve the quality and safety of health care, stimulating a broad array of stakeholders to engage in the quality-improvement effort [1]. Numerous studies before and since have documented the quality problems that pervade the United States health care system, including the underuse, overuse, and misuse of interventions and other errors in care [2–4]. These problems are found in all types of services (ie, preventive, acute, chronic), patient age groups, treatment settings, managed and unmanaged care, and somatic and behavioral health services. The result has been a health care system in which Americans are guaranteed, at best, a 50% chance of receiving the care they need when they need it. Although general quality improvements have occurred during the last several years, enormous differences persist between the performance of the health care system as a whole and the top

This article was supported by multiple contracts and grants from the Robert Wood Johnson Foundation (grant #48021), the US Department of Veterans Affairs (contract #101-G67214/101-G67215), UPMC For You, Highmark Foundation, Staunton Farm Foundation, FISA Foundation, with matching support from the Centers for Medicare and Medicaid.

*Corresponding author. E-mail address: keyser@rand.org (D.J. Keyser).

0193-953X/08/$ – see front matter
doi:10.1016/j.psc.2007.11.002

10% of health plans that report on quality [5]. As the National Committee for Quality Assurance (NCQA) points out in its latest report, *The State of Health Care Quality 2006*, "These 'quality gaps' represent the continuing failure to consistently deliver care in accordance with well-established guidelines and exact a substantial toll in terms of both lives and economic costs" [5].

In its second report, *Crossing The Quality Chasm: A New Health System for the 21st Century* (2001), the IOM explained that quality problems occur typically because of fundamental shortcomings in the ways care is organized and proposed a framework for fixing the system based on six aims for high-quality health care (Box 1) [6] and 10 rules to guide system redesign (Box 2) [6]. The report also identifies several critical pathways for systems change, including adopting new ways of delivering care; making effective use of information technologies; managing the clinical knowledge and skills of the workforce; developing effective teams and coordinating care across patient conditions, services, and settings; improving how health care quality is measured; and adopting payment methods that create incentives for and reward good quality. Such changes have implications for multiple levels of the health care system: (1) the interactions between patients and their individual clinicians; (2) the functioning of small units of care delivery ("microsystems"), such as interdisciplinary teams or staff located on inpatient units; (3) the functioning of organizations that house the microsystems; and (4) the environment of policy, payment, regulation, accreditation, and similar external factors that shape the environment in which health care organizations deliver care [7].

Box 1: The six aims of high-quality health care

High-quality health care should be
Safe: Avoiding injuries to patients from the care that is intended to help them

Effective: Providing services based on scientific knowledge to all who could benefit and refraining from providing services to those not likely to benefit (avoiding underuse and overuse, respectively)

Patient-centered: Providing care that is respectful of and responsive to individual patient preferences, needs, and values and ensuring that patient values guide all clinical decisions

Timely: Reducing waits and sometimes harmful delays for both those who receive and those who give care

Efficient: Avoiding waste, including waste of equipment, supplies, ideas, and energy

Equitable: Providing care that does not vary in quality because of personal characteristics such as gender, ethnicity, geographic location, and socioeconomic status

From: Committee on Quality of Health Care in America, Institute of Medicine. Crossing the quality chasm: a new health system for the twenty-first century. Washington, DC: National Academies Press; 2001. p. 5–6; with permission. Copyright © 2001, National Academy of Medicine.

Box 2: The Quality Chasm's 10 rules to guide the redesign of health care

1. Care based on continuous healing relationships
2. Customization based on patient needs and values
3. The patient as the source of control
4. Shared knowledge and the free flow of information
5. Evidence-based decision making
6. Safety as a system property
7. The need for transparency
8. Anticipation of needs
9. Continuous decrease in waste
10. Cooperation among clinicians

From: Committee on Quality of Health Care in America, Institute of Medicine. Crossing the quality chasm: a new health system for the twenty-first century. Washington, DC: National Academies Press; 2001. p. 8; with permission. Copyright © 2001, National Academy of Medicine.

When the second IOM report was released, questions were raised regarding the applicability of the Quality Chasm framework for improving health care for mental health/substance use conditions. Mental health/substance use conditions are pervasive, frequently intertwined, and, when left untreated, can result in devastating consequences. More than 33 million Americans are treated annually for these conditions, including 20% of all working adults (18–54 years of age) [8] and 21% of adolescents [9]. Millions more have reported that they needed treatment for mental health/substance use conditions but did not receive it [9–11]. Unipolar major depression and alcohol use are the second and fourth leading sources of disease burden in established market economies, following ischemic health disease (first) and cardiovascular disease (third), respectively [12]. Unipolar depressive disorders, alcohol use disorders, schizophrenia, and bipolar affective disorder also are among the top five leading causes of years of life lived with disability in 15- to 44-year olds [13].

Recognition of the prominent role that mental and substance use health care plays in the overall health care system led a range of key stakeholders, foundations, and national agencies to charge the IOM with exploring the implications of the Quality Chasm for the field of mental health and addictive disorders and identifying the barriers and facilitators to achieving significant improvements along the six aims of health care quality. The IOM convened a special Committee on Crossing the Quality Chasm: Adaptation to the Mental Health and Addictive Disorders (the Committee), which produced a new IOM report entitled *Improving the Quality of Health Care for Mental and Substance Use Conditions* (2006) [14]. The findings and conclusions of this report, its implications for psychiatrists in their daily practice, and recommendations for changes in public policy are summarized in a recent article by Pincus and colleagues [15] in the *American Journal of Psychiatry*.

This article describes the two major phenomena that shaped the Committee's overall findings and informed its overarching recommendations for improving the quality of health care for mental health/substance use conditions. These phenomena are (1) the co-occurrence of mental health, substance use, and general health conditions and (2) differences in mental/substance use health services delivery compared with general health care. It then offers several examples of national and local efforts currently underway that are addressing these differences and have the potential for achieving significant quality improvements in mental/substance use health care delivery and outcomes.

CO-OCCURRENCE OF MENTAL HEALTH, SUBSTANCE USE, AND GENERAL HEALTH CONDITIONS

One of the Committee's overall findings is that mental, substance use, and general illnesses are highly interrelated, especially with respect to chronic illness and injury [16,17]. The rates of co-occurrence of mental health and substance use conditions are high, estimated at 15% to 40% [18–20]. They also accompany a substantial number of chronic illnesses, such as cancer, diabetes, and heart disease [16]. Forty percent to 56% of individuals who have mental illness have a clinically significant general medical condition. Mental health/substance use conditions also are associated with the leading causes of outpatient visits, including headache, fatigue, and pain. Because mental health/substance use conditions seem similar to other somatic problems, they may go undetected in the general health settings where they are seen most often.

This high level of comorbidity is not without consequences. Mental/substance use illnesses significantly compromise the treatment outcomes for general health conditions. For example, 20% of heart attack patients suffer from depression, tripling their risk of death. The disabilities and other adverse effects resulting from mental health/substance use conditions also impose an enormous cost on society [21]. Mental health/substance use conditions are the fifth most expensive category of health care conditions in the United States among individuals not residing in nursing homes or other institutions [22]. Direct spending for mental/substance use health care by all health care purchasers in the United States totaled an estimated $104 billion in 2001 (82% for mental illnesses and 18% for substance use illnesses), representing 7.6% of all health care spending [23]. Additional costs related to mental/substance use illnesses, such as secondary health problems, loss of productivity in the workplace, and social problems requiring the involvement of the welfare and criminal and juvenile justice systems are even higher.

Given these circumstances, the Committee concluded that improving care delivery and health outcomes for mental health, or for substance use, or for general health conditions depends on improving the care delivery and outcomes for the other two types of conditions. Therefore, the first overarching recommendation of the Committee with respect to improving the quality of health care for mental health/substance use conditions states: "Health care for general, mental, and substance-use problems and illnesses must be delivered with an understanding of the inherent interactions between the mind/brain and the rest of the body."

DIFFERENCES IN THE DELIVERY OF SERVICES FOR MENTAL HEALTH/SUBSTANCE USE COMPARED WITH GENERAL HEALTH CARE

The Committee also found that health care for mental health/substance use, like general health care, often is ineffective, not patient-centered, untimely, inefficient, inequitable, and at times unsafe, and that it, too, requires fundamental redesign. A review of all peer-reviewed studies published between 1992 and 2000 assessing the quality of care for many different clinical conditions found that only 27% of the studies reported adequate rates of adherence to established, evidence-based practice guidelines [24]. Subsequent studies continue to document clinicians' departures from evidence-based practice guidelines for conditions as varied as attention deficit hyperactivity disorder [25], anxiety disorders [26], comorbid mental and substance use illnesses [27], depression in adults [28] and children [29], opioid dependence [30], and schizophrenia [31].

According to the NCQA, mental health presents a disturbing exception to the overall pattern of health care improvement during the last several years: "The quality of care for Americans with mental health problems remains as poor today as it was several years ago. Patients on antidepressant medication are about as likely to receive appropriate care today as they were in 1999. Similarly, patients hospitalized for mental illness are only marginally more likely to receive appropriate follow-up care" [5].

Furthermore, as stated previously, many individuals who need treatment receive none [9–11]. Although recent studies have shown some improvements in access to and receipt of care, especially among those who have the most severe mental illnesses [8,10] and depression [32], and among children [33], access for those who have less severe mental illnesses [10] and for ethnic minorities [8] has declined. Less is also known about errors in or injuries caused by treatment for mental and substance use conditions than in general health care [34,35].

The Committee further determined that the Quality Chasm recommendations for the redesign of health care are as applicable to mental/substance use health care as they are to general health care. The second overarching recommendation of the Committee for improving the quality of health care for mental and substance use conditions states: "The aims, rules, and strategies for redesign set forth in *Crossing the Quality Chasm* should be applied throughout mental/substance use care on a day-to-day operational basis but tailored to reflect the characteristics that distinguish care for these problems and illnesses from general health care." This recommendation recognizes the importance of a number of characteristics that are unique to mental and substance use health care, including obstacles to patient-centered care; weaknesses in the infrastructure for measurement and improvement; poor linkages across mental health, substance use, and general health; lack of involvement in the National Health Information Infrastructure; insufficient workforce capacity for quality improvements; and a differently structured marketplace. These problems are summarized briefly below.

Obstacles to Patient-Centered Care

In the original Quality Chasm report, patient-centered care (ie, care that respects and responds to patient preferences, needs, and values) is identified as one of the six aims of quality health care. In mental and substance use health care, however, residual stereotypes, including patients' inability to exercise their capacity for decision making, potential for dangerousness, and perceptions of drug dependence as solely volitional, result in stigma and discrimination by health care providers and in public policy. These adverse consequences on patients' ability to exercise their capacity for decision making can seriously impede self-management of their illnesses and limit the prospects for recovery, particularly when patients are coerced into treatment.

Weak Measurement and Improvement Infrastructure

The infrastructure needed to measure, analyze, publicly report, and improve the quality of mental and substance use health care is less well developed than that for general health care. For example, clinical assessment and treatment practices are not yet standardized and classified for use in administrative datasets. In addition, although reliable and valid instruments exist, performance measurement for mental/substance use health care has not received sufficient attention in either the private or public sectors, and outcome measurement (ie, measurement-based care) is not applied widely. Finally, quality improvement methods are not yet permeating day-to-day operations, and effective strategies often are not used to disseminate advances.

Poor Linkages Across Mental Health, Substance Use, and General Health

Mental health and substance use health services typically remain separated from each other and from general health care. For the most part, society continues to rely on the education, child welfare, and other non–health care sectors to deliver mental/substance use care, and the specialized services that are needed by individuals who have more severe illnesses are located in public-sector programs apart from the private sector. These disconnected care delivery arrangements require multiple provider handoffs of patients for different services and the transmission of information to and joint planning by all of these providers, organizations, and agencies, but accountability for this coordination is unclear.

Lack of Involvement in the National Health Information Infrastructure

Although major public- and private-sector collaborations are underway to develop the critical components of a National Health Information Infrastructure (eg, electronic health records with decision support for clinicians; a secure platform for exchanging patient information across health care settings; data standards so that shared information will be understandable to all users), to date, the involvement of mental health/substance use care in these efforts has been limited. The field also is falling behind in related health information technology initiatives. In 2004, the Agency for Health Care Research and Quality awarded $139 million in grants and contracts to promote the use of health information technology. Health care for mental/substance use conditions was strongly not represented among either the applicants or awardees. Of the nearly 600 applications for funding, only "a handful" had any substantial behavioral health component, and of the 103 grants awarded, only one specifically targeted health care for mental health and substance use [14].

Insufficient Workforce Capacity for Quality Improvement

Several factors limit the quality and capacity of the mental and substance use workforce. First, there is much greater variation in the education and training of the workforce in mental/substance use health care than in other areas of health care. This variation results in part from a number of across-the-board deficiencies in education (eg, the lack of any "core knowledge" across disciplines about substance use) and from variations in licensure, credentialing, and continuing education. Second, the high prevalence of unconnected solo practices among mental health and substance use care providers impedes the adoption of information technology, the widespread use of evidence-based practices, and other advances in care. Finally, most of the workforce is inadequately prepared to use the Internet and other communication technologies that have the potential to enhance service delivery.

Differently Structured Marketplace

The mental health and substance use health care marketplace is distinguished by the dominance of government (both state and local) purchasers, frequent purchase of insurance for mental/substance use health care separately from other health care (ie, "carve-out" arrangements), the tendency of private insurance to avoid covering or to offer more limited coverage to individuals who have mental and substance use illnesses, and government purchasers' greater use of direct provision and purchase of care rather than insurance arrangements.

NATIONAL AND LOCAL EFFORTS FOR IMPROVING THE QUALITY OF MENTAL/SUBSTANCE USE HEALTH CARE

In the face of these complexities, it is clear that innovative approaches to quality improvement in the arena of mental health/substance use need to be developed and implemented by multiple stakeholders at all levels of the health care system. Among the numerous recommendations put forth by the Committee are strategies for bridging knowledge gaps about treatment, the effectiveness of care delivery, and mechanisms and processes for improving quality in routine clinical practice as well as across the diverse clinicians, organizations, and systems delivering mental/substance use health care. Addressing these knowledge gaps also will require changes in public policy related to the purchasing, management, and delivery of mental health/substance use care that are applicable at all levels, including patients and families, microsystems of care, health care organizations, and the larger health care environment [7].

Although the scope of required change is daunting in its entirety, a range of quality improvement efforts currently underway exemplify the types of approaches that might be pursued to bring mental/substance use health care quality to the level of clinical effectiveness that evidence shows is possible. A few examples of such efforts are described briefly in the following sections.

Depression in Primary Care: Linking Clinical and System Strategies
Funded by The Robert Wood Johnson Foundation, Depression in Primary Care: Linking Clinical and System Strategies has sought to increase the use of effective models for treating depression in primary care settings [36]. This $12 million national program was developed to address three issues: (1) depression is a serious and prevalent chronic disease that should be conceptualized in a way that is parallel to other chronic conditions (eg, asthma and diabetes); (2) longitudinal approaches to the treatment of depression as a chronic illness are effective but currently are not implemented by health systems and practitioners; (3) putting these approaches into place requires a combination of strategies targeting clinical and economic systems at multiple levels, engaging patients/consumers, providers, practices, plans, and purchasers.

Start-up activities for this program began in July 2000. To date, the program has funded eight incentive grants (demonstration projects), 26 value research grants, and four targeted leadership grants. Direction and technical assistance have been provided by The Department of Psychiatry, University of Pittsburgh School of Medicine.

The incentive grants have supported partnerships comprised of health practice/delivery systems, health insurance plans, managed behavioral health organizations, pharmacy benefit managers, and academic institutions that are involved in primary care delivery for patients 18 years of age or older. Because of the disincentives created by the differently structured marketplaces for mental and substance use health care, the goal of these partnerships was to demonstrate the implementation of an effective clinical model of quality improvement accompanied by the changes in incentives and organizational arrangements necessary to support the clinical model. The goal was to create a decision-making environment that encourages evidence-based, cost-effective treatment of depression by harmonizing the incentives for primary care physicians to treat depression with the incentives for treating other conditions.

The value research grants supported creative and innovative research projects focused on developing, implementing, and documenting the value of combined clinical and economic/system strategies for improving the treatment of depression in primary care. Some of the value grants, for example, developed new approaches for measuring clinical outcomes; others implemented innovative strategies for creating incentives for providers, practices, and health plans to improve their clinical information systems. In combination, these grants addressed a number of the problems associated with the existing weak infrastructure for assessment and measuring quality improvement in mental and substance use health care.

The targeted leadership grants supported leadership development within primary care medical specialties, with a particular focus on emerging physicians with an interest in and commitment to studying and treating depression as a chronic disease.

Program Evaluation of Mental Health Services in the Veterans Health Administration of the Department of Veterans Affairs

In August 2006, the Office of Policy, Planning, and Preparedness of the Department of Veterans Affairs (VA) contracted with the Altarum Institute (Ann Arbor, Michigan) and the RAND-University of Pittsburgh Health Institute to conduct a formal program evaluation of the mental health services for schizophrenia, bipolar disorder, posttraumatic stress disorder, major depression, and substance use disorders in the Veterans Health Administration (VHA).

Using the structure-process-outcomes model of health care quality, the study addresses three overarching questions:

1. What services are available to veterans (eg, type/level of staffing, hours of operation, availability of evidence-based practices)?
2. What services do veterans receive (eg, extent to which evidence-based practices are implemented, frequency and timing of services)?
3. Do the services make a difference (eg, patient satisfaction, quality of life, functional status)?

The information required to answer these questions is being collected from four different sources: existing administrative data; a formal survey of the VA Medical Centers; a client survey of a sample of veterans who received care for the five targeted mental health diagnoses from the VHA and a sample of veterans who received care for the same diagnoses (with the exception of substance use disorder) outside the VA; and abstraction of medical records for veterans who are VHA users.

A key component of this evaluation has been the development of a set of fully specified performance indicators for the five targeted mental health diagnoses that can be used to assess the degree to which VA program outcome goals are being met.

An initial step in this process was to categorize the proposed set of performance indicators according to the level of evidence supporting the link between the performance indicator and the desired program outcome. Level I indicators were either evidence based or similar to those developed by expert or national organizations and had the highest level of evidence; level II indicators were not evidence based but were developed by consensus views and guidelines of professional organizations or experts; level III indicators were broadly endorsed by relevant stakeholders but had no firm evidence of a process-outcome link.

Second, an assessment was made of the adequacy of the proposed program outcome goals and related performance indicators for evaluating the effectiveness of program results and the efficiency of service delivery. Primary emphasis was placed on ensuring optimal alignment of VA goals for health care and VHA program outcomes with the critical outcomes of health care as formulated by the IOM's Quality Chasm Report, the President's New Freedom Commission *Report on Mental Health* [37], and the VA Mental Health Strategic Plan [38]. Recognizing the IOM's six aims for high-quality care as the industry standard [6,14], an expanded set of indicators was developed that described effectiveness, safety, patient-centeredness and recovery, timeliness, efficiency, and equity.

Based on a literature review, expert consultations, and careful analysis of existing sets of clinical practice guidelines, additional steps were then taken to (1) identify an exhaustive pool of relevant level I performance indicators; (2) generate a new set of level II performance indicators including key guideline-recommended processes of care not described by existing level I performance indicators; and (3) generate a new set of level III performance indicators, including key IOM domains or VA Mental Health Strategic Plan priorities not described by existing level I or level II performance indicators.

Next, in consultation with a VA Clinical Advisory Group, a core set of level I and level II performance indicators was identified as being robust, valid, and a VA priority. Operational definitions then were developed for each performance indicator, including the identification of data sources that efficiently provide the information necessary to populate the indicators.

Finally, using existing strength-of-evidence and strength-of-recommendation rating systems, each performance indicator was classified according to the strength of its process-outcome link.

The complete set of indicators and methods is intended to serve as a template for VA, state, and local mental health and substance use disorders systems and for other major health care stakeholders for monitoring and improving the quality of care for serious mental illness.

Bridging the Silos of Medicaid Managed Care: a Community-Based Quality Improvement Collaborative for Enhancing the Delivery of Care for Maternal Depression

The goal of this 3-year community-based quality improvement initiative is to improve access to and engagement in evidence-based treatment services for maternal depression among at-risk pregnant women or mothers who are enrolled in the HealthChoices Program in Allegheny County, Pennsylvania. The work emanates from a broader region-wide effort to improve maternal and child heath care policy and practice in Allegheny County, the results of which underscored a sentinel issue related to both maternal depression and other priority areas of health care: how to bridge the existing silos between physical and mental health care systems to provide the quality of care that is needed [39,40]. This initiative uses Medicaid managed care as a vehicle for bridging these silos and uniting policymakers, health plans, providers, programs, and patients in a coordinated effort to enhance service delivery for maternal depression among the target population. It is funded by a consortium of local foundations with matching support provided by the Centers for Medicare and Medicaid Services.

Building on and integrating existing systems and resources, the collaborative partners are designing a local adaptation of the Chronic Care Model [41] for treatment of maternal depression in Allegheny County. The key components of the initiative are organized around that model's six strategies for change, many of which explicitly address the problems associated with mental and substance use health care. These strategies include

1. Mobilizing community resources to meet patients' needs
2. Creating a culture, organization, and mechanisms that promote safe, high-quality care
3. Empowering and preparing patients to manage their health and health care
4. Assuring the delivery of effective, efficient clinical care and support in self management
5. Promoting clinical care that is consistent with scientific evidence and patient preferences
6. Organizing patient and population data to facilitate efficient and effective care

These strategies have been operationalized through the development and implementation of evidence-based protocols for screening pregnant women and mothers in primary care settings for maternal depression, determining their risk level based on the results of the screening, and effectively managing their care as they move between primary care and mental health settings. Care managers at the physical health managed care organizations serve as the primary point of contact for the primary care and mental health providers, and agreed-upon processes for information sharing are being established among all parties. Providers also are being trained on how to engage patients in more effectively the care process, with a particular focus on providing service and treatment options that better meet their patients' needs, values, and preferences. Other relevant community organizations (eg, family support centers, nurse-family partnerships, and in-home service providers, among others) will be engaged in the care delivery process as needed.

The demonstration began in the fall of 2007 and is scheduled to end in the spring of 2010. The expected outcomes include a set of policy and health system infrastructure supports for effectively adapting and sustaining the Chronic Care Model for treatment of maternal depression in Allegheny County and throughout the Pennsylvania HealthChoices Program; documented improvements in specific health care processes (eg, screening, engagement in treatment, longitudinal follow-up) that are critical to the successful treatment of depression; and potentially longer-term contributions to society through positive overall health outcomes for at-risk mothers and children and related reductions in health care disparities.

SUMMARY

The work of the Committee on Crossing the Quality Chasm: Adaptation to the Mental Health and Addictive Disorders and the resulting IOM report *Improving the Quality of Health Care for Mental and Substance Use Conditions* represent another important milestone along the road to improving the quality of United States health care. Although it remains unclear to what extent this second call for action by the IOM will result in significant improvements in the quality of the mental/substance use health care system over either the short or long term, the steps taken to date by a wide range of stakeholders in the behavioral health field suggest that the system is poised for change. As the profession ventures into the new health environment of the twenty-first century, two things are certain. First, the field of mental and substance use health care will need to work in a coordinated and collaborative fashion with the rest of medicine, and vice versa. Second, to be successful, the Quality Chasm framework for systems improvement must be adapted to the special features of the mental health and substance use system.

References

[1] Cohn LT, Corrigan JM, Donaldson MS, editors. To err is human: building a safer health system. Washington, DC: National Academies Press; 2000.
[2] Schuster ME, McGlynn EA, Brook RH. How good is the quality of health care in the United States? Milbank Quarterly 1998;76(4):517–63.
[3] Chassin MR, Galvin RW. The urgent need to improve health care quality. JAMA 1998;280(11):1000–5.
[4] McGlynn EA, Asch SM, Adams J, et al. The quality of health care delivered to adults in the United States. N Engl J Med 2003;348:2635–45.
[5] National Committee for Quality Assurance. The state of health care quality 2006. Washington, DC: National Committee for Quality Assurance; 2007.
[6] Institute of Medicine. Crossing the quality chasm: a new health system for the twenty-first century. Washington, DC: National Academies Press; 2001.
[7] Berwick D. A user's manual for the IOM's "Quality Chasm" report. Health Aff 2002;21(3): 80–90.
[8] Kessler RC, Demler O, Frank RG, et al. Prevalence and treatment of mental disorders, 1990 to 2003. N Engl J Med 2005;352:2515–23.
[9] Substance Abuse and Mental Health Services Administration. Results from the 2003 National Survey on Drug Use and Health: national findings. DHHS Publication #SMA 04-3964, NSDUH Series H-25. Rockville (MD): Substance Abuse and Mental Health Services Administration; 2004.
[10] Mechanic D, Bilder S. Treatment of people with mental illness: a decade-long perspective. Health Aff 2004;23:84–95.
[11] Wu L-T, Ringwalt CL, Williams CE. Use of substance abuse treatment services by persons with mental health and substance use problems. Psychiatr Serv 2003;54(3):363–9.
[12] Murray CJ, Lopez AD. The global burden of disease: a comprehensive assessment of mortality and disability from diseases, injuries and risk factors in 1990 and projected to 2020. Global Burden of Disease and Injury Series, vol. I. Cambridge (MA): Harvard School of Public Health; 1996.
[13] World Health Organization. The world health report 2001–Mental health: new understanding, new hope. Geneva, Switzerland: World Health Organization; 2001.
[14] Institute of Medicine Committee on Crossing the Quality Chasm: adaptation to mental health and addictive disorders. Improving the quality of health care for mental and substance use conditions. Washington, DC: National Academies Press Report; 2006.

[15] Pincus HA, Page AEK, Druss B, et al. Can psychiatry cross the quality chasm? Improving the quality of health care for mental and substance use conditions. Am J Psychiatry 2007;164: 712–9.

[16] Katon W. Clinical and health services relationships between major depression, depressive symptoms, and general medical illness. Biol Psychiatry 2003;54:216–26.

[17] Kroenke K. Patients presenting with somatic complaints: epidemiology, psychiatric co-morbidity and management. Int J Methods Psychiatr Res 2003;12(1):34–43.

[18] Grant BF, Stinson FS, Dawson DA, et al. Prevalence and co-occurrence of substance use disorders and independent mood and anxiety disorders: results from the National Epidemiologic Survey on Alcohol and Related Conditions. Arch Gen Psychiatry 2004;61:807–16.

[19] Grant BF, Stinson FS, Dawson DA, et al. Co-occurrence of 12-month alcohol and drug use disorders and personality disorders in the United States: results from the National Epidemiologic Survey on Alcohol and Related Conditions. Arch Gen Psychiatry 2004; 61:361–8.

[20] Horvitz-Lennon M, Kilbourne A, Pincus HA. From silos to bridges: meeting the general health care needs of adults with severe mental illnesses. Health Aff 2006;25:659–70.

[21] Frank RG, McGuire TG. Economics and mental health. In: Cuyler AJ, Newhouse JP, editors. Handbook of health economics, vol. 1B, No. 17. Amsterdam: Elsevier Science B.V.; 2000. p. 893–954.

[22] Thorpe KE, Florence CS, Joski P. Which medical conditions account for the rise in health care spending? Health Aff 2004; Web exclusive (W4):437–45. Available at: http://contenthealthaffairs.org/cgi/content/full/hlthaff.w4.437/DC1. Accessed August 20, 2007.

[23] Mark TL, Coffey RM, Vandivort-Warren R, et al. U.S. spending for mental health and substance abuse treatment, 1991–2001. Health Aff 2005;24:w133–42. Available at: http://content.healthaffairs.org/cgi/content/full/hlthaff.w4.437/DC1. Accessed August 15, 2007.

[24] Bauer MS. A review of quantitative studies of adherence to mental health clinical practice and guidelines. Harv Rev Psychiatry 2002;10(3):138–53.

[25] Rushton JL, Fant K, Clark SJ. Use of practice guidelines in the primary care of children with attention-deficit hyperactivity disorder. Pediatrics 2004;114:e23–8.

[26] Stein MB, Sherbourne CD, Craske MG, et al. Quality of care for primary care patients with anxiety disorders. Am J Psychiatry 2004;161:2230–7.

[27] Watkins K, Burnam A, Kung F, et al. A national survey of care for persons with co-occurring mental and substance use disorders. Psychiatr Serv 2001;52:1062–8.

[28] Simon GE, Von Korff M, Rutter C, et al. Treatment processes and outcomes for managed care patients receiving new antidepressant prescriptions from psychiatrists and primary care physicians. Arch Gen Psychiatry 2001;58:395–401.

[29] Richardson L, Di Guiseppe D, Christakis DA, et al. Quality of care for Medicaid-covered youth treated with antidepressant therapy. Arch Gen Psychiatry 2004;61:475–80.

[30] D'Aunno T, Pollack HA. Changes in methadone treatment practices: results from a national panel study. JAMA 2002;288:850–6.

[31] Buchanan RW, Kreyenbuhl J, Zito JM, et al. The schizophrenia PORT pharmacological treatment recommendations: conformance and implications for symptoms and functional outcome. Schizophr Bull 2002;28:63–73.

[32] Olfson M, Marcus SC, Druss B, et al. National trends in the outpatient treatment of depression. JAMA 2002;287(2):203–9.

[33] Glied S, Cuellar AE. Trends and issues in child and adolescent mental health. Health Aff 2003;22(5):39–50.

[34] Bates DW, Shore MF, Gibson R, et al. Examining the evidence. Psychiatr Serv 2003;54: 1–5.

[35] Moos RH. Iatrogenic effects of psychosocial interventions for substance use disorders: prevalence, predictors, prevention. Addiction 2005;100:595–604.

[36] Depression in Primary Care: Linking Clinical and System Strategies. Available at: http://www.depressioninprimarycare.org. Accessed August 24, 2007.

[37] President's New Freedom Commission on Mental Health: Final Report to the President. Available at: http://mentalhealthcommission.gov/reports/reports.htm. Accessed August 30, 2007.

[38] Department of Veterans Affairs. A Comprehensive VHA Strategic Plan for Mental Health Services-Revised. VHA Mental Health Strategic Plan Workgroup/Mental Health Strategic Health Care Group, Office of the Assistant Deputy Under Secretary for Health, July 9, 2004.

[39] Pincus HA, Thomas SB, Keyser DJ. Improving maternal and child health care: a blueprint for community action in the Pittsburgh region. MG-225-HE. Santa Monica (CA): RAND Corporation; 2005.

[40] Building a model maternal and child health care system in the Pittsburgh region: a community-based quality improvement initiative. Santa Monica (CA): RAND Corporation; 2006.

[41] Improving Chronic Illness Care: The Chronic Care Model. Available at: http://www.improvingchroniccare.org/index.php?p=The_Chronic_Care_Model&s=2. Accessed August 30, 2007.

Psychiatr Clin N Am 31 (2008) 57–72

PSYCHIATRIC CLINICS
OF NORTH AMERICA

ELSEVIER
SAUNDERS

Quality Outcomes Management: Veterans Affairs Case Study

Subhash C. Bhatia, MD[a,b,*], Praveen P. Fernandes, MD[a,b]

[a]Mental Health and Behavioral Sciences Department (116A), VA Nebraska–Western
Iowa Health Care System, 4101 Woolworth Avenue, Omaha, NE 68105, USA
[b]Department of Psychiatry, Creighton University, 3528 Dodge Street,
Omaha, NE 68131, USA

S ince July 1930, the Veterans Administration has had the privilege to provide medical care and other services to honorably discharged veterans.
The foundation for support of these services is embodied in the quote
from President Abraham Lincoln: "To care for him who shall have borne
the battle, and for his widow and his orphan." To elevate the level of service
to all those who paid the price for freedom, in 1989 the status of the Veterans
Administration was raised to the cabinet level under the name Department of
Veterans Affairs (VA). This department included the Veterans Health Administration (VHA) and the Veterans Benefit Administration (VBA).

VETERANS AFFAIRS CASE STUDY
In the 1970s and 1980s, the VHA primarily provided hospital-based acute care
and had a reputation of delivering poor quality, substandard care. VA hospitals
were often viewed as "dangerous, dirty and scandal-ridden" [1].

Under the leadership of Dr. Kenneth W. Kizer [2], Under Secretary Health,
the VA developed a reform proposal, the "Vision for Change," and translated
it into the "Prescription for Change." This proposal provided the road map for
structural and functional changes in the VHA to enhance the quality of care
and steer the VHA toward efficiency and excellence.

Under this plan, administrative structural changes were made and 22 Veterans
Integrated Service Networks (VISNs) created. Each VISN had a leadership team
of a director and a medical director supported by a staff for finance and quality
management. Most VISNs had about 10 hospitals, 25 to 30 ambulatory clinics,
four to seven nursing home care units, and one to three domiciliary care
programs. Before this change, the VA was structured on a regional basis.

*Corresponding author. Department of Psychiatry, Creighton University, 3528 Dodge Street,
Omaha, NE 68131. E-mail address: subhash.bhatia@va.gov (S.C. Bhatia).

0193-953X/08/$ – see front matter   Published by Elsevier Inc.
doi:10.1016/j.psc.2007.11.006   psych.theclinics.com

This change also resulted in creation of the patient care service lines (PCSLs), extended care and rehabilitation, imaging, primary care and specialty medicine, mental health, pathology and laboratory medicine, and surgery and specialty medicine. Each PCSL has a leadership team of a director, medical director, executive nurse, and executive administrator. The PCSL leadership, with the support of leaders from various facilities, is responsible for strategic planning, enhancing quality of care and safety, and meeting the financial goals set by the VISN leadership. PCSLs are also responsible for implementing new initiatives and mandates from the VA headquarters.

Also under Dr. Kizer's [3] proposed plan, two significant operational changes were implemented. The first was an all-electronic health information system, which included a computerized patient records system (CPRS), veterans heath information system and technology architecture (VistA) imaging, bar-code medication administration (BCMA), and My HealtheVet. The second operational change was quality of care enhancement, achieved by having high-value performance measures from several quality dimensions and domains such as prevention indices, chronic disease management, and palliative care. Since then, the VHA has actively used these performance measures and tracked and monitored them for effectiveness. Over time, these measures have grown significantly in number and have been designated as critical for performance and are used for leadership performance incentives.

These changes have transformed the quality of VA heath care; consequently, the VHA has received accolades from health care industry leaders. The news media has taken note of this improvement as well. In a 2005 edition of the *Washington Monthly*, VHA's care was described as "the best care anywhere" [1]. Adam Oliver, Academic Fellow at London School of Economics Health and Social Care, titled his publication in the *Milbank Quarterly* as, "The Veterans Heath Administration: an American success story?" of a public sector organization [4]. He stated that, "some evidence shows that its overall performance now exceeds that of the rest of US health system."

Because of the technological innovations and their positive impact on quality of VA health care, in 2006 the VA received the prestigious "Innovations in American Government Award" from the Ash Institute for Democratic Governance and Innovation at Harvard University's John F. Kennedy School of Government [5], specifically for innovations with the VistA information system.

A 2005 RAND Corporation study [6] found that for 6 straight years, the VHA outperformed on 294 measures of quality in disease prevention and treatment in comparison with all other sectors of American health care.

Peer-reviewed publications, the *New England Journal of Medicine* [7] and *Archives of Internal Medicine* [8], also validated the VHA's provision of higher quality of care compared with community providers.

These achievements are due to the implementation of changes driven by the will of the VA leadership and its commitment and adherence to its professed mission, vision, and core values (Box 1).

Box 1: Modal description of the Veterans Affair's mission, vision, and core values

- Mission—dedication to health care needs of veterans through quality patient care, education, and research
- Vision—recognition as a provider of choice for veterans, a leader in delivery of quality health care, dedication to providing accessible health care, and being an employer of choice
- Core values—commitment, compassion, excellence, respect, and trust

---

These are all being achieved while adhering to principles of sound management practices as well as factoring in growth and cost effectiveness. The VHA is also committed to cultivation of a culture of continuous quality improvement and a focus on patient safety.

The VA has expanded the definition of value of the services it provides, as to the relationship of quality to cost. Each of the value domains (Fig. 1) is objectively defined and measurable [9]. The measurements serve as the basis for performance improvements and accountability. The domain of cost effectiveness in the VHA is also a value equation between the first three domains and cost.

At present, the "new VA" operates 153 major medical centers and 880 clinics serving over 1 million patients a week [10]. It has 15,000 physicians, 33,000 other health care providers, 61,000 nurses, 25,000 affiliated faculty physicians, 90,000 trainees, and 140,000 volunteers [10] who pride themselves in delivering high-quality, superb care. Recently, Dr. Perlin [11], Under Secretary of Health, Department of Veterans Affairs, in his farewell massage stated that, "VHA is recognized as Gold Standard." He also stated that, "the *New York Times*, the *Washington Post*, the *Washington Monthly*, *Business Week*, and *US News and World Report* all have lauded VHA as a model health care system, efficiently providing 'the best care any where'" [1,12,13]. *Time Magazine*, in its article, "How VA Hospitals Became the Best?" [14], also acknowledged the VA's improved delivery of health care.

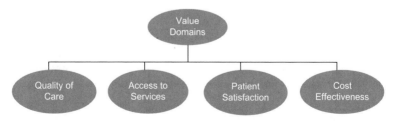

Fig. 1. An overview of the VA's value domains. (*Data from* Perlin JB, Kolodner RM, and Roswell RH. The Veterans Health Administration: quality, value, accountability, and information as transforming strategies for patient-centered care. Am J Manag Care 2004; 10(11 Pt 2):828–36.)

The changes that transformed the "old VA" into today's VA and its impact on mental health care delivery are described below.

DEPARTMENT OF VETERANS AFFAIRS TECHNOLOGY AND QUALITY OF CARE

On the basis of Dr. Kizer's vision for change, information technology professionals, in collaboration with VHA clinicians, in 1996 developed the CPRS, a Windows-based user interface with VistA. VistA has over 100 programs that support day-to-day clinical, administrative, and financial functions. The price of maintaining the CPRS is approximately $87/patient/year [5]. This is less than the cost of unnecessary duplication of a medication or a laboratory test. In addition to the CPRS, the information system has VistA imaging, the BCMA, and My HealtheVet.

This electronic health record system enables clinicians to view health records, including laboratory and imaging data, at any of the more than 1400 VA clinical care sites. When veterans move from one geographic location to another and access their care at another VA site, they have the benefit of portable electronic health records. This obviously promotes continuity of care.

The value of this system became apparent for the 40,000 veterans who were the victims of Hurricane Katrina and who subsequently left the New Orleans, Louisiana, and Gulfport, Mississippi, areas. If there were only paper VA records, these would have been destroyed and patients would have needed new sets of evaluations and assessments. Availability of electronic health records allowed veterans to access appropriate timely care at another VA site and eliminated unnecessary and costly duplication.

It is reported that availability of integrated electronic health records prevents one in five patient's unnecessary laboratory studies and one in seven unnecessary hospitalizations. A report by the Institute of Medicine [15] and the *American Journal of Medical Quality* [16] underscored the need for use of information technology to improve patient safety and to saves lives.

Physician electronic order entry for medication, laboratory tests, and consultations reduces ordering errors. Also, when nurses administer medications after verifying two patient-specific identifiers as validated by the BCMA system, medication administration errors are reduced. Nationally, 3% to 8% of prescriptions have errors, whereas the VA's accuracy rate for prescriptions is reported to be greater than 99.997% [13].

My HealtheVet is designed for veterans accessing care in the VA and is their personal health journal. The patient is able to enter information about his or her own health, including records of laboratory values. This system is also linked to federal and VA benefits and other resources that allow veterans to order their prescription refills on line. The system is secure and allows the veteran control as to who has access to this information.

The VistA imaging system can store and archive radiology, ultrasound, endoscopy, pathology slides, dermatology lesion images, and EKG wave forms. These images are combined with the text data.

In a 1995 pharmacy reform to reduce geographical variability in the use of medications, the VA established the National Pharmacy Benefit Management package. The use of pharmaceuticals in the VA and community is similar. Also, the pharmacy software package alerts care providers to drug interactions, which reduces medication- related complications and thereby unwarranted hospitalizations.

Finally, but no less important, electronically legible patient health records have a significant hand-off value for surrogate providers during after hours, weekends, and holidays. Availability of integrated medical information reduces redundant duplication of procedures and cost of care.

ACCESS TO CARE AS A MEASURE OF QUALITY

In the VA, the dictum "access delayed is access denied" is given special attention. To prevent long delays in accessing care, the VHA has implemented advanced clinical access (ACA). The principles of the ACA model are to remove constraints and barriers for access to care, increase throughput, and adhere to best practices in efficiency to promote models of care [17]. The goal of this initiative is to provide same-day service.

The ACA initiative—originally a tool to improve access to primary and specialty care clinics—has now spread to other service areas of the VHA: inpatient flow and administrative ACA and management. As of 2007, access and efficiency improvement initiatives are now encompassed under the title of "systems redesign."

Box 2 illustrates some key principles of systems redesign as they apply to mental health in the VA.

THE DEPARTMENT OF VETERANS ADMINISTRATION MENTAL HEALTH

As a part of Dr. Kizer's prescription for change, positive changes in mental health service delivery paralleled those in medicine and surgery.

In 1997, VA's Mental Health Strategic Health Care Group stated, "Each eligible (enrolled) veteran will have access to comprehensive, integrated continuum of high quality effective mental health services by the year 2002" [18].

The mental health program guidelines [18] also described principles for (1) organizing mental health care, (2) program planning, (3) providing quality mental health care, and (4) individual patient treatment planning. The program manual also provides guidance for special populations of veterans with the following:

- Seriously mentally ill
- Substance use disorder
- Posttraumatic stress disorder
- Homeless mentally ill
- Elderly with psychogeriatric disorders
- Veterans living in rural areas
- Women and minority veterans

Box 2: Key principles of systems redesign

Balancing demand and supply

This is the first step, as an imbalance between demand and supply will predictably lead to a backlog and waits and delays for patients. Measurement of external demand (demand from the outside), internal demand (demand created by providers, as in the case of return appointments), and supply (as in appointment slots or clinic time) helps to determine whether they are in balance. If not, changes are made to create a balance, in the process working down and preventing a backlog. These changes are the following:

Shaping demand: decreasing internal demand by decreasing the frequency of clinically justified revisits. Providers are encouraged to avoid routine scheduling and attempt to spread out appointments when clinically appropriate.

Increasing capacity: extending revisit intervals can significantly open up a clinic's capacity. Using alternatives to traditional clinical visits, such as telephone encounters to check on side effects or decide on dosage adjustments, allows clinic slots to be used for patients who need to come in. Another process for improving capacity is discharging stable patients to primary care. As the majority of VA patients have a primary care provider, stable patients (not symptomatic and no change in medication for 6 months or longer) can be referred back to them for continuing care for refill of prescriptions. This graduation of stable patients to primary care allows a mental health clinic's capacity to be used for sicker patients.

Decreasing no-show rates

No-shows are a waste of a clinic's capacity and add to the rework of scheduling another appointment from future clinical capacity. The VA subsumes no-show rates under the broader performance measure of "missed opportunity rate," which is a combination of no-show rates and rates of cancellation by clinic or by patient after the time of appointment. The target for this combined performance measure for mental health is 16%. Steps to reduce no-show rates include an automated phone reminder system, letter reminder, and personal calls by clinic or volunteer staff. Negotiating a date and time for the next visit with the patient is often helpful, as is discussing the clinical reason for the patient to show up for the next visit and a reminder to cancel if he or she cannot make it.

Implementing service agreement with primary care

Service agreements are a written agreement between primary care and mental health to benefit workload reduction of both clinical services. A service agreement can require that primary care try first-line antidepressants like serotonin-reuptake inhibitors for treating simple depression and anxiety before deciding to refer patients to mental health. The service agreement can additionally require that primary care take over the management of stable patients from mental health, with the definition of stability mutually agreed on. Mental health service, in return, assures primary care of a prompt consult appointment without delay.

For details on each of these elements, refer to the *VHA Program Guide 1103.3* [18].

Mental health programs in the VHA have not benefited only by Dr. Kizer's vision, but also by the VHA's mental health leadership. One of the significant decisions by this leadership was adoption and implementation of the president's "New Freedom Commission Report on Mental Health" [19]. The general summary of the six goals in this report, which are adopted under action agenda of the VHA, [20] include the following:

> To understand that mental health is essential to overall health. Mental illness is the leading cause of overall disability in the United States, and there is a need to dispel the stigma of mental illness and need for collaborative care with other providers.
>
> To ensure that mental health care is consumer and family driven. The care plan should be individualized and customized in full partnership with the patient, and should include a component of family education.
>
> To eliminate disparities in mental health services by improving access to humane, culturally competent quality mental health care for all ages in all geographic areas.
>
> To screen veterans for psychiatric and co-occurring substance use disorders in primary care settings across the life span, followed by full assessment and referral for appropriate services.
>
> To achieve excellence in mental health care delivery through accelerated research and to use this research for recovery, resilience, and, ultimately, for prevention and cure for mental illnesses.
>
> To use technology for integrated electronic health care records and personal information and to use telehealth consultations to promote coordinated continuum of mental health care.

Currently, these goals are embodied in the comprehensive VHA mental health strategic plan [21].

In the VHA there is increasing focus on mental health. At present, the VA is the largest provider of mental health services in the United States, with an annual budget of $3 billion. Mental health services are provided in each of the 153 medical centers and 882 outpatient clinics. The VA now offers telemental health services at 164 community-based outpatient clinics (CBOCs) and 89 medical centers. In addition, 23 sites support home telemental health. During fiscal year 2006, 20,000 veterans with mental health needs received consultations through the VA's telemental health network. The VA also operates 80 hospital-based mental health programs that focus on Operation Enduring Freedom (OEF) from Afghanistan and Operation Iraqi Freedom (OIF), in collaboration with 200 specialized posttraumatic stress disorder (PTSD) programs and more than 150 general mental health clinics [22].

To promote safety for mental health patients, on August 16, 2007, the VHA launched a Mental Health Center of Excellence at Canandaigua, VA Medical Center, New York, as well as a National Suicide Prevention Hot Line: 1-800-273-TALK (8255). The service in Spanish can also be obtained at 1-888-628-9454.

In addition, the VA has 10 mental illness research, education, and clinical centers with the following focus areas:

- Causes of serious mental illness
- Schizophrenia
- Post-deployment mental illness
- Bringing research into practice
- Psychotic disorders
- PTSD and Alzheimer's disease
- Schizophrenia
- PTSD and dementia
- Suicide prevention
- Comorbid conditions and mental illness
- Comorbid substance use disorders

The VHA is one of the largest contributors to education of medical students, residents, and other health care practitioners in all health care fields, including mental health.

COMPREHENSIVE, SEAMLESS CONTINUUM OF VETERANS AFFAIRS MENTAL HEALTH SERVICES

Consistent with the president's "New Freedom Commission Report on Mental Health," the VHA is committed to patient-centered, comprehensive, and seamless continuum of quality psychiatric and substance use disorder services for all ages and in all geographic areas while maximizing the use of technology. The VHA provides continuum of mental health services through a variety of settings (ie, hospital, residential, ambulatory, and community-based care) [15]. Box 3 lists the specific settings where these services are delivered.

Recently, the VA launched the RANGE MHICM for rural and small markets. By the end of October 2006, 13 VISNs took advantage of this initiative to establish 14 new RANGE MHICM programs.

There has also been significant emphasis on integration of mental health in primary care and mental health care for the veterans returning from OEF (Afghanistan) and OIF (Iraq) war theaters. OEF/OIF programs, through their outreach efforts, also address the mental health needs during pre- and post-deployment phases.

In addition, on the basis of the second recommendation of the president's "New Freedom Commission Report on Mental Health," the VHA has adopted recovery-oriented approach to mental health care. As a part of this initiative, peer support programs and mental health consumer councils are being established and are part of the mental health strategic plan in every VISN. Through mental health consumer councils, the consumers of mental health services through programs like vet-to-vet or peer-to-peer or peer technician provide input to improve the quality of mental health care and to provide support to veterans to overcome mental illness and substance use disorder. The goals of these councils are to dispel stigma, to instill optimism, and to propagate

Box 3: Mental health service centers

- Psychiatric intensive care unit for inpatient care
- Nursing home extended care units
- Psychiatric residential rehabilitation program for step-down and step-up care
- Substance abuse residential rehabilitation program
- Domiciliary and day hospital
- Mental health intensive case management (MHICM) patterned after the assertive, community treatment
- Rural access network for growth enhancement (RANGE), a rural MHICM
- Mental health clinic
- PTSD clinical team and co-occurring substance use and PTSD treatment teams
- Home-based telemental health as well as palliative care
- Community residential care
- Substance use disorder day program
- Intensive outpatient and outreach programs
- Compensated work therapy
- Vocational rehabilitation and community-based veterans centers

In addition, at various sites nationally there are specialized programs (ie, military sexual trauma treatment, gambling addiction, eating disorder, and sexual addiction).

the recovery message to the mentally ill. These peer support programs in the VA are growing in numbers nationally.

INFORMATION TECHNOLOGY AND MENTAL HEALTH

The VA's CPRS is programmed to generate alerts and performance reminders for clinicians about screens such as for depression, PTSD, and tobacco and alcohol use disorders in primary and specialty care clinics, as well as about performance measures for preventive, chronic disease and palliative care. CPRS reminders help with successful implementation of best practices related to depression screen [23]. Elder depression care in the primary care clinics helps to reduce mortality [24]. These screens allow timely and early detection and prompt intervention. It is generally well accepted that early detection and management of depression in primary care settings not only reduce mortality, but also reduce cost of medical care and enhance the quality of life of veterans and their families.

Some of the alerts related to mental health include tobacco use screens, timely monitoring of newly implemented metabolic side effects of antipsychotic drugs, and 90-day continuity-of-care measures for substance use disorder patients that are based on research findings that good addiction outcomes are contingent on adequate length of treatment [25,26]. In addition, alerts for timely completion of Abnormal Involuntary Movement Scale are included as movement disorders are a side effect of antipsychotic therapy. Also, completion of the Global Assessment of Function scale adds value to quality and measurement of effectiveness of mental health interventions.

To provide a safe work and patient care environment in the VA, VHA Directive 2003-048 [27] provides guidance to establish patient record flags (PRFs). PRFs serve as an advisory to immediately alert care providers or designated staff to know about patients with risk of violence. There are two categories of PRFs: category I Behavioral National and category II Local. Category I Behavioral National PRFs are for patients with a history of repeated acts or credible threats of violence against patients or staff at the VA, possession of weapons, suicidal or parasuicidal behavior within the health facility, repeated disruptive behavior, or sexual harassment of patients or staff. The Category II Local PRFs are established by the VISN or local facilities for patients who are drug seekers or in research protocols. PRFs are not used to punish or discriminate against patients or to merely enhance staff convenience. There are processes in place to evaluate removal of these PRFs every 2 years.

When a patient with PRFs accesses care and the provider opens the electronic health records, the first window that opens is for the alert related to the PRF. This violence prevention plan in the VHA is consistent with the safe environment of care by the Joint Commission [28].

Integrated health information that includes an updated problem list, availability of vital signs, medical/surgical history, and laboratory and imaging data allows mental health care providers to see mind–body interaction and treat the individual holistically. This allows safe interventions.

The CPRS can also develop provider-specific or evidenced-based clinical care templates like evidenced-based alcohol screening [29]. In addition, the CPRS can be programmed to interface with voice recognition software that gives providers the options to type or dictate their clinical care notes, thereby saving time and reducing transcription costs. This also allows ready access to most up-to-date information to surrogate providers.

Providers can also access the most recent literature (eg, the *New England Journal of Medicine* and other publications). Information from these publications can be incorporated into the medical records to support provider's clinical decisions.

In addition, because of this integrated national database, clinicians and researchers have access to a large data warehouse to test clinical hypotheses or to engage in prospective or retrospective studies with the power of big numbers. This can contribute significantly to best practices in the field.

One such recent study, in light of the 2006 U.S. Food and Drug Administration Advisory Committee recommendation for black-box warning based on an association between selective serotonin reuptake inhibitors (SSRIs) treatment and suicide, was evaluated by Gibbons and Associates [30] in a naturalistic study on 226,866 veterans who received a diagnosis of depression and were treated with SSRIs or other antidepressants. Contrary to the Advisory Committee's findings, the results showed SSRIs as having a protective effect against suicide. This large study population obviously lends credence to such findings. Similarly, in a study at 17 VA medical centers, Rosenheck and colleagues [31] demonstrated the comparability of haloperidol, a first-generation antipsychotic, with olanzapine, an atypical antipsychotic drug but at a lower cost associated with haloperidol. In another large-scale study, Greenberg and Rosenheck [32] studied the value of Global Assessment of Function scale measurements for mental health care outcomes in the VA.

Because of the national connectivity capability of telepsychiatry equipment, a recently commissioned multisite cooperative research to study long-acting injectable risperidone in treatment of schizophrenia used centralized videoconferencing telepsychiatry assessment by expert raters to reduce inter-rater variability of assessments between research subjects.

INTEGRATION OF MENTAL HEALTH INTO PRIMARY CARE

In this model, mental health care providers such as psychiatrists, psychologists, psychiatric social workers, clinical chaplains, and clinical nurse practitioners are embedded into the primary care clinical teams. This integration is intended to increase access to mental health care, especially for those patients who feel stigmatized about going to mental health programs. Also, the mental health specialist can (1) provide brief and rapid assessment and brief bio-psychosocial interventions, (2) educate the primary care providers and staff in management of uncomplicated psychiatric disorders, (3) provide education about health psychology, and (4) facilitate referral of complex patients to specialty mental health programs.

The mental health provider also supports the primary care providers in screening for depression, PTSD, alcohol use disorder, and smoking cessation while assisting the primary care provider with chronic pain management, adaptation to and coping with acute and chronic illness, working through losses, enhancing social and interpersonal skills, anger management, cardiac risk reduction, and compliance with recommended medications and recommended treatment services.

The mental health provider can provide curbside consultations or traditional consultation and liaison services. These mental heath interventions are known to reduce mortality, decrease cost of medical and surgical care, and improve quality of life of veterans and their families.

Availability of telemedicine connection to distant sites allows patients from isolated rural communities and remote areas to access needed mental health services. The VHA has established CBOCs in areas with relatively smaller population centers. The primary purpose of these clinics is to bring the services closer to where patients are so as to not force them to drive long distances, especially in rural states such as in VISN 23 (the Dakotas, Nebraska, Iowa, and Minnesota). With long driving distances, both the time and the cost of gasoline present barriers for patients to access health care services. All these sites have telemedicine equipment connected with the medical centers, and patients are frequently assessed through the use of this system. These and other rural health initiatives by the VHA enhance access and reduce disparities to care.

It is now mandated that all eligible veterans with mental health care needs will have access to emergent, urgent, and routine care and that no

Box 4: Mental health performance measures

Access

Enhanced access to mental health services in CBOCs with enrollment of more than 1500 uniques

Improved access for homeless veterans to mental health, substance use disorders, primary care intake clinics, programs, and adequate follow-up

Access by at least 4% of patients in psychosis registry to the MHICM [34]

Reduced waiting time for new and established patients for clinic appointments; patients requesting services must be seen within 14 days

Reduce missed opportunity rates as they apply to patients who are no-shows or whose appointments have been cancelled by the clinic or by the patient after the appointment time. All no-show patients are contacted to ensure that they are safe and to educate them about the value of their calling in to accommodate patients who are waiting.

Healthy community

Seamless transition for severely ill/seriously injured based on information from the Department of Defense before military discharge to be contacted by the VA case manger within 7 days for services

Timely (within 24 hours) independent attending note on all inpatient admissions and evidence of involvement by the attending care provider for day-to-day care of inpatients (a resident supervision measure)

Quality

Annual screening for alcohol misuse. AUDIT-C, three questions, four points each score based on the frequency and amount of drinking. A score of 4 in men and 3 in women; range, 0–12, is considered positive [35,36].

Substance use disorder–90-day continuity of care. Applies to all patients in treatment for substance use disorder except those in opioid substitution. This measure is based on the research finding that duration of treatment is a factor most consistently associated with successful treatment outcome for addictive disorders [25,26].

Annual four "yes/no" questions PTSD screening in primary clinics. Have you ever had any experience that was so frightening, horrible, or upsetting that in the last month you have:

Had any nightmares about it when you did not want to?

Tried hard not to think about it or went out of the way to avoid situations that remind you of it?

Been constantly on guard, watchful, or easily startled?

Felt numb or detached from others, activities, or your surroundings?
Three "yes" answers is a positive screen [37].
Annual depression screening using PH-Q2. These two questions are scored on three points each. A total score of 3 or more is a positive depression screen. The two questions asked are the following: During the last 2 weeks how often have you been bothered by any of the following? (1) Little interest or pleasure in doing things, and/or (2) feeling down, depressed, or hopeless [38].

(continued on next page)

Box 4 (*continued*)

New diagnosis of depression (no history of depression during prior 120 days or no antidepressant prescription during the prior 90 days of index episode of depression). The patient may be in primary care or mental health programs. Successful measure requires (1) optimal practitioner contacts of at least three follow-up practitioner contacts during 12 weeks, one of which must be with a prescribing practitioner and the other two (may include telephone contacts) with eligible providers, and (2) optimal medication coverage for at least 84 days from index prescription date [39].

Smoking screening and cessation of smoking measures. These measures are scored on (1) offered medication to assist with cessation, (2) provision of brief counseling and offered referral, and (3) tobacco use during the past 12 months (lower is better).

Satisfaction

This measure is for inpatient and outpatient care, with a question about overall satisfaction about quality of care. The responses are excellent, very good, good, fair, or poor. Positive scores are considered to be very good or excellent. The survey is aimed to capture a patient's perceptions about the following:

• Access

• Coordination of health care

• Courtesy and dignity

• Education about health care

• Emotional support

• Involvement of family and friends

• Patient preferences about health care decisions

• Smooth transition between inpatient and outpatient care

• Continuity of care

• Timely and appropriate pharmacy services and specialist care

• In addition, there is an expectation about strategic workforce planning, leadership and employee development, diversity management, employee satisfaction, and Equal Employment Opportunity management

Cost effectiveness

The VA's enabling goal is to deliver world-class service to veterans and their families by applying sound business principles that result in effective management of people, communication, technology, and governance.

patient will have to wait for more than 14 days for assessment and intervention.

THE DEPARTMENT OF VETERANS ADMINISTRATION QUALITY PERFORMANCE MEASURES FOR MENTAL HEALTH

The Office Quality and Performance [33] has various performance measures under various domains. The ones relevant to mental health are shown in Box 4.

SUMMARY

During the last decade, the VA has made major strides in enhancing quality of medical, surgical, and mental health care for veterans. This has been accomplished through the will and commitment of VHA leadership by changes in the administrative structure (eg, creating VISNs and PCSLs; use of state-of-the-art technology for electronic health records, implementation of high-value preventative and chronic disease management performance measures, and the ability to track their effectiveness).

Parallel with these changes, the quality of mental heath care in the VA has also improved, as have mental health education and research. Implementation of the president's "New Freedom Commission Report on Mental Health" on mental health added further momentum toward quality enhancement. Implementation of comprehensive, seamless continuum of care for the seriously mentally ill and recovery-oriented intervention strategies are helping to enhance the VA's ability to help reintegrate mentally ill veterans into the society.

In addition, in light of the recent wars and greater need for mental health services, there has been increased focus on mental health, leading to enhancement of resources specifically for OEF (Afghanistan) and OIF (Iraq) veterans, PTSD, and traumatic brain injury care. The VA is currently one of the largest providers of mental health services in the nation.

The use of telemental health technology, establishment of CBOCs, use of advanced clinical access tools, and integration of mental health into primary care have been successful in improving access to mental health care.

In addition, depression, PTSD, and alcohol-related screens in primary care have significant potential for early diagnosis and prompt intervention. This certainly will improve outcomes for these disorders. Having mental heath providers embedded in the primary care teams will also support early recognition and intervention. This integration can reduce the cost of medical and surgical care and improve outcomes and quality of life for veterans and their families.

Acknowledgments
The authors thank Rowen K. Zetterman, MD, Chief of Staff, VA Nebraska–Western Iowa Health Care System and Professor of Departments of Internal Medicine and Section of Gastroenterology, University of Nebraska Medical Center, for thoughtful review and comments to improve the quality of this article.

References
[1] Longman P. The best care anywhere. Washington Monthly 2005; January/February: 37–48.
[2] Kizer KW. Vision for change. A plan to restructure the Veterans Health Administration. Washington, DC: Department of Veterans Affairs; 1995.
[3] Kizer KW. The "new VA": a national laboratory for health care quality management. Am J Med Qual 1999;14(1):3–20.
[4] Oliver A. The Veterans Health Administration: an American success story? Milbank Q 2007;85(1):5–35.
[5] Department of Veterans Affairs-VistA: Winner of Innovations in American Government Award. Presented by the Ash Institute for Democratic Governance and Innovation at Harvard University, John F. Kennedy School of Government, Washington, DC; July 10, 2006.

[6] RAND Corporation. Improving quality of care—how the VA outpaces other systems in delivering patient care. Research highlights 2005. Available at: http://www.rand.org/pubs/research_briefs/RB9100/index1.html. Accessed December 28, 2007.

[7] Jha AK, Perlin JB, Kizer KW, et al. Effect of the transformation of the Veterans Affairs Health Care System on the quality of care. N Engl J Med 2003;348(22):2218–27.

[8] Asch SM, McGlynn EA, Hogan MM, et al. Comparison of quality of care for patients in the Veterans Health Administration and patients in a national sample. Ann Intern Med 2004;141:938–45.

[9] Perlin JB, Kolodner RM, Roswell RH. The Veterans Health Administration: quality, value, accountability, and information as transforming strategies for patient-centered care. Am J Manag Care 2004;10(11 Pt 2):828–36.

[10] Prepared remarks by: the Honorable R James Nicholson, Secretary Department of Veterans Affairs to American Legion National Convention at Reno, Nevada, August 29, 2007. Available at: http://www.alacrastore.com/storecontent/voxantcq/2007tr08290003s99. Accessed January 06, 2008.

[11] Perlin JB. VHA recognized as "Gold Standard." A farewell message 2006. Available at: http://www.usminstitute.org/spotlights/sp20.html. Accessed December 28, 2007.

[12] Stein R. VA care is rated superior to that in private hospitals. Washington Post January 20, 2006;A4. Available at: http://www.washingtonpost.com/wp-dyn/content/article/2006/01/19/AR2006011902936.html. Accessed December 28, 2007.

[13] Arnst C. The best medical care in the US: how veterans affairs transformed itself—and what it means to rest of us. Bus Week July 17, 2006. Available at: http://www.businessweek.com/magazine/content/06_29/b3993061.html. Accessed December 28, 2007.

[14] Waller D. How VA hospitals became the best? Time 2006;168(10):36. Available at: http://www.time.com/time/magazine/article/0,9171,1376238,00.html.   Accessed December 28, 2007.

[15] Committee on Quality of Healthcare in America, Institute of Medicine. Crossing the quality chasm. A new health system for 21st century. Washington, DC: National Academy Press; 2001.

[16] Weir CR, Hicken BL, Rappaport HS, et al. Crossing the quality chasm: the role of information technology departments. Am J Med Qual 2006;21(6):382–93.

[17] Armstrong B, Levesque O, Perlin JB, et al. Reinventing Veterans Health Administration: focus on primary care. Healthc Q 2006;9(2):80–5.

[18] Department of Veterans Affairs. VHA Program Guide 1103.3. Mental Health Program Guidelines "for the new Veterans Health Care Administration." Office of the Patient Care Services Mental Health Strategic Group (116). Veterans Health Administration Washington, DC 20420, June 3, 1999.

[19] President's New Freedom Commission on Mental Health Report. Achieving the promise: transforming America's mental health care system. United States Department of Health and Human Services. July 22, 2003. Available at: http://www.mentalhealthcommission.gov/reports/FinalReport/toc.html. Accessed December 28, 2007.

[20] Department of Veterans Affairs, Action Agenda. Achieving the promise: transforming mental health care in VA. Veterans Health Administration. December 1, 2003. Available at: http://www.va.gov/oig/54/reports/VAOIG-06-03706-126.pdf.   Accessed December 28, 2007.

[21] Department of Veterans Affairs. Comprehensive VHA mental health strategic plan, aligned with the recommendations of the Action Plan. Washington, DC: Veterans Health Administration. May 2, 2005. Available at: ftp://vaww.mentalhealth.med.va.gov/main/vha_mh_strategic_plan.pdf. Accessed January 02, 2008.

[22] Remarks by: the Honorable R. James Nicholson, Secretary of Veterans Affairs, at National Mental Health Meeting. Alexandria (VA), July 16, 2007. Available at: http://www.washingtonpost.com/wp-srv/nation/document/walter-reed/nicholson_transcript_07107.html. Accessed January 02, 2008.

[23] Kirkcaldy RD, Tynes LL. Depression screening in a VA primary care clinic. Psychiatr Serv 2006;57(12):1694–6.

[24] Gallo JJ, Bogner HR, Morales KH, et al. The effect of a primary care practice-based depression intervention on mortality in older adults: a randomized trial. Ann Intern Med 2007;146(10):689–98.

[25] Crits-Christoph P, Siqueland L. Psychosocial treatment for drug abuse: selected review and recommendations for national health care. Arch Gen Psychiatry 1996;53(8):749–56.

[26] Finney JW, Moos RH. Psychosocial treatment for alcohol use disorders. In: Nathan PF, Gorman JM, editors. A guide to treatments that work. 2nd edition. New York: Oxford University Press; 2002. p. 157–68.

[27] Department of Veterans Affairs. National Patient Records Flags. VHA Directive 2003–048. Dated August 28, 2003. Available at: http://www1.va.gov/vhapublications/ViewPublication.asp?pub_ID=277.html. Accessed December 28, 2007.

[28] Environment of care guide book. JCAHO 1997. Available at: http://www.jointcommission.org/NR/rdonlyres/8912113B-72C6-409F-82A9-77F187424C34/0/07_bhc_npsgs.pdf. Accessed January 06, 2008.

[29] Bradley KA, Williams EC, Achtmeyer CE, et al. Implementation of evidence-based alcohol screening in the Veterans Heath Administration. Am J Manag Care 2006;12(10):597–606.

[30] Gibbons RD, Brown CH, Hur K, et al. Relationship between antidepressants and suicide attempts: an analysis of the Veterans Health Administration data sets. Am J Psychiatry 2007;164(7):1044–9.

[31] Rosenheck R, Perlick D, Bingham S, et al. Effectiveness and cost of olanzapine and haloperidol in the treatment of schizophrenia: a randomized controlled trial. JAMA 2003;290(20):2693–702.

[32] Greenberg GA, Rosenheck RA. Use of nationwide outcome monitoring data to compare clinical outcomes in specialized mental health programs and general psychiatric clinics in the Veterans Health Administration. Psychiatr Q 2006;77(2):151–72.

[33] Department of Veterans Affairs performance measurement system including JCAHO hospital core measures. Office of Quality and Performance (10 Q) July, 2007.

[34] Plan for enhancing deployment of intensive case management for severely mentally ill. Memorandum (10N-1-22) from the Assistant Deputy Under Secretary to VISN Directors. Available at: http://www.oqp.med.va.gov/cpg/PSY/G/TM/Secion1Measure1.doc. Accessed December 28, 2007.

[35] Bradley KA, Kivlahan DR, Zhou XH, et al. Using alcohol screening results and treatment history to assess the severity of at-risk drinking in Veterans Affairs primary care patients. Alcohol Clin Exp Res 2004;28(3):448–55.

[36] Dawson DA, Grant BF, Stinson FS, et al. Effectiveness of the derived Alcohol Use Disorders Identification Test (AUDIT-C) in screening for alcohol use disorders and risk drinking in the US general population. Alcohol Clin Exp Res 2005;29(5):844–54.

[37] Breslau N, Peterson EL, Kessler RC, et al. Short screening scale for DSM-IV posttraumatic stress disorder. Am J Psychiatry 1999;156(6):908–11.

[38] Williams JW Jr, Mulrow CD, Kroenke K, et al. Case-finding for depression in primary care: a randomized trial. Am J Med 1999;106(1):36–43.

[39] VA/DOD clinical practice guideline for management of major depression in adults. Available at: http://www.oqp.med.va.gov/cpg/MDD/MDDBase.htm. Accessed August 30, 2007.

Psychiatr Clin N Am 31 (2008) 73–84

PSYCHIATRIC CLINICS
OF NORTH AMERICA

ELSEVIER
SAUNDERS

Incorporating the Prevention Paradigm into Administrative Psychiatry

Michael T. Compton, MD, MPH[a,b,*]

[a]Department of Psychiatry and Behavioral Sciences, Emory University School of Medicine, Atlanta, GA, USA
[b]Department of Family and Preventive Medicine, Emory University School of Medicine, Atlanta, GA, USA

MENTAL ILLNESS PREVENTION AND MENTAL HEALTH PROMOTION

Administrative psychiatry has much to gain from the prevention paradigm. This overview describes some of the ways that administrative psychiatry would benefit from incorporating the principles of mental illness prevention and mental health promotion. Mental illness prevention centers on reducing risk factors and enhancing protective factors to decrease the incidence and prevalence of various psychiatric illnesses, to prevent or delay recurrences of mental illnesses, and to alleviate the impact of these illnesses on affected persons, their families, and society [1,2]. As such, mental illness prevention encompasses the clinical, community, and policy strategies designed to reduce the burden of mental illnesses, preferably by intervening well before illness onset [3]. Mental health promotion aims to impact determinants of mental health so as to increase positive mental health, reduce inequalities, build social capital, create health gain, and narrow the gap in health expectancy between countries and groups [2,4]. Mental health promotion includes strategies that support resiliency, enhance psychosocial functioning, and protect against the development of mental illnesses [3].

Several federal initiatives have highlighted the utility of prevention in psychiatry. The landmark 1994 Institute of Medicine report entitled *Reducing Risks for Mental Disorders: Frontiers for Preventive Intervention Research*, which was mandated by the US Congress to review the field of prevention science, describes the advances in knowledge about risk and protective factors related to mental and behavioral disorders as well as the development of evidence-based interventions addressing such factors [1]. *Healthy People 2010*, which is a set of health

This work was supported by grant #MH067589 from the National Institutes of Health.

*Emory University School of Medicine, 49 Jesse Hill Jr. Drive, S.E., Room #333, Atlanta, GA 30303. *E-mail address*: mcompto@emory.edu

0193-953X/08/$ – see front matter
doi:10.1016/j.psc.2007.11.004

objectives for the nation to achieve during the present decade, addresses several prevention concerns in mental health domains, such as reducing the suicide rate, increasing the number of persons seen in primary health care who receive mental health screening and assessment, and increasing the proportion of juvenile justice facilities that screen new admissions for mental health problems [5]. The US Preventive Services Task Force, an independent panel of experts in primary care and prevention that systematically reviews the evidence and develops recommendations for clinical preventive services, has provided guidelines related to mental health regarding screening for such conditions as alcohol misuse, dementia, depression, drug abuse, and suicide risk [6]. The recent *President's New Freedom Commission on Mental Health* recognized that early detection and treatment of mental illnesses are critical [7]. The Substance Abuse and Mental Health Services Administration maintains the National Registry of Evidence-Based Programs and Practices, which catalogues substance abuse and mental health preventive interventions [8]. Therefore, psychiatric administrators have a number of guidelines and recommendations readily available to promote a prevention orientation within their broad missions, which often include overseeing clinical services and programs, educating and training future psychiatrists and other mental health professionals, supporting research, and participating in the public arena through community consultation and advocacy.

HISTORICAL CONTEXT OF THE PREVENTION PARADIGM IN PSYCHIATRY

Considerations of prevention in the mental health professions have a long and rich history. Although the organization and financing of mental health services now are determined largely by marketplace-driven forces such as managed care and pharmaceuticals rather than by federally sponsored community mental health efforts, it is important for administrators to appreciate the historical developments in the prevention paradigm. Prevention was an important theme of the community mental health movement of the 1960s. The President's Commission on Mental Health convened during the Carter administration emphasized the relevance of prevention for mental health policy [9]. More recently, the report of the New Freedom Commission on Mental Health during the Bush administration [7] strongly recommended continued efforts aimed at suicide prevention and pointed out model early-intervention programs such as the Nurse-Family Partnership, which is focused on nurses intervening during pregnancy to prevent mental health problems in childhood [10]. That report also recommended implementing empirically supported prevention and early-intervention approaches at the school district, local school, classroom, and individual student levels, reflecting the fact that much of the work of prevention is done in nonclinical settings.

Although the fervor for prevention in the 1960s has a long-lasting legacy, and prevention continues to be suggested as holding much unrealized promise, a thorough review of the key historical events in the evolution of prevention in psychiatry is beyond the scope of this overview. This history is provided in the aforementioned Institute of Medicine report [1]. Whereas the community mental health movement of the 1960s may have been overly optimistic with respect to prevention [11], the mental health promotion/mental illness prevention paradigm of today is a research-based discipline, cognizant of its limitations but poised to bring renewed hope to practitioners, researchers, and policy-makers alike [3].

A BRIEF OVERVIEW OF TWO CLASSIFICATIONS OF PREVENTION

Like other chronic medical conditions, mental illnesses can be considered from the perspective of prevention in addition to treatment. Given the level of disability and functional impairment (eg, psychosocial dysfunction, loss of productivity, decrements in disability-adjusted life-years) associated with a number of serious psychiatric illnesses and substance use disorders [12], pursuing prevention goals is particularly relevant for psychiatry. The importance of prevention, however, has traditionally been overlooked in the context of psychiatric disorders [13] in comparison to other disease categories, such as infectious diseases and, more recently, chronic medical conditions such as diabetes mellitus and cardiovascular disease. Indeed, many psychiatrists and allied mental health professionals with whom administrative psychiatrists interact may be largely unaware of the ways in which a prevention paradigm can promote mental health and reduce the burden of psychiatric and addictive disorders. Incorporating a preventive approach—the consideration of risk and protective factors, epidemiologic data, evidence-based preventive interventions, health promotion, and cost-effectiveness—within psychiatry can be called "prevention psychiatry" [9].

Prevention has been classified traditionally in terms of primary, secondary, and tertiary prevention [9,14]. Primary prevention involves the application of health promotion or specific protective interventions that modify risk factors to reduce the incidence of the disease or condition in question. For example, primary prevention of cardiovascular disease includes efforts to promote cessation of cigarette smoking. In turn, primary prevention of cigarette smoking includes means to restrict accessibility to cigarettes, taxation of tobacco products, and regulations against advertisements directed toward youth. In psychiatry, one aspect of the primary prevention of major depression, for example, may entail efforts to reduce adverse childhood events, which are known risk factors for the later development of depression [15]. Secondary prevention includes screening, early identification, and treatment of incipient illnesses that may be in a latent stage before symptomatic presentation. An example in general medicine is the use of mammography to detect breast cancer in very early stages, an intervention that is associated with decreased morbidity and mortality. Secondary prevention also is applicable to psychiatric disorders. For example, increasing interest is being focused on secondary prevention of schizophrenia by reducing treatment delays through early detection and intervention efforts [16]. Other secondary prevention efforts target the effective treatment of childhood disorders and trauma. For example, timely and effective supportive therapy for childhood physical and sexual abuse—an alarmingly common set of risk factors for a multitude of adverse physical and psychiatric outcomes—bolsters self-esteem and consequently reduces risk of depression in adulthood. Tertiary prevention consists of minimizing the morbidity and mortality of an established illness. Tertiary prevention may be accomplished by preventing relapse, comorbidity, psychosocial disability, and functional impairment. Much of the treatment that physicians provide, both in general medicine and psychiatry, can be considered tertiary prevention.

In addition to the traditional primary, secondary, and tertiary prevention categories, preventive interventions also can be classified according to the population to which an intervention is targeted [1], termed "universal," "selective," and "indicated" preventive interventions. A universal intervention is applied to the population in general. For example, fluoridation of the water supply, iodination of salt, and childhood vaccinations are classic examples of universal interventions in public health and general medicine. An example in psychiatry is public service announcements or media campaigns designed to prevent substance abuse [9]. Many universal interventions (eg, standards for prenatal care, fortification of foods with essential vitamins) have broad effects on health in many domains, and detecting an effect on the incidence of a particular disorder may be difficult because nonspecific interventions may be adopted by society before their specific role in preventing specific illnesses can be established [17].

The next type of preventive intervention in the newer classification scheme, which also would fall within the primary prevention category of the traditional classification (Fig. 1), is a selective intervention. A selective intervention targets a specific subgroup, a subset of the population experiencing a specific risk factor. Thus, individuals who have hyperlipidemia are targeted for more intensive screening and treatment to avert coronary heart disease and other cardiovascular complications. In the mental health field, interventions that target youth who are at elevated risk for delinquency, conduct disorder, or substance abuse by virtue of the presence of specific risk factors would be considered selective preventive interventions.

An indicated intervention is applied to an even smaller group of individuals who are at particularly high risk. Indicated interventions are often positioned at the boundary between the traditional primary and secondary forms of prevention, or they may be considered synonymous with secondary prevention (see Fig. 1). That is, there is some conceptual overlap between indicated interventions that target individuals at high risk for the future development of the disease and secondary prevention efforts that screen for and detect latent disease during the presymptomatic stage. Secondary prevention typically refers to screening/detection efforts, whereas an indicated intervention is, in fact, an intervention that is meant to reduce the likelihood of disease onset in a screened/detected high-risk group. In general medicine, an example of an indicated preventive intervention is aspirin chemoprevention in patients at

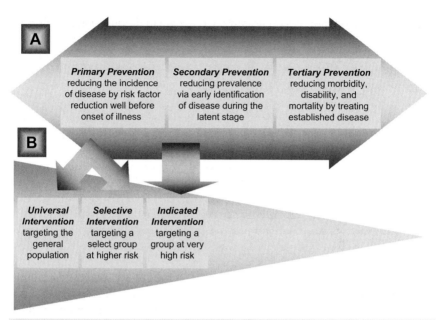

Fig. 1. Two classifications of prevention. (A) The traditional classification of primary, secondary, and tertiary prevention, based on the stage of disease during which the intervention is applied. (B) The newer classification of universal, selective, and indicated preventive interventions, defined by the target population to which the intervention is directed. As shown by the arrows, primary prevention usually is accomplished through universal and selective preventive interventions. Indicated preventive interventions are often at the border between primary and secondary prevention.

high risk for coronary heart disease by virtue of the presence of many risk factors, not just older age. Indicated preventive interventions in psychiatry are exemplified by recent efforts to identify and treat individuals who are at ultra-high risk for schizophrenia although they do not yet meet the criteria for the diagnosis [16]. Durlak and Wells [18] reviewed 130 indicated preventive intervention mental health programs for children and adolescents and found that behavioral and cognitive-behavior programs for children who had subclinical disorders are as effective as psychotherapy for children who have established problems and that there is substantial evidence for the effectiveness of programs targeting incipient externalizing problems that customarily are the least amenable to change once they reach clinical status. The 1994 Institute of Medicine report elaborates on the application of these types of preventive interventions to a number of psychiatric illnesses and substance use disorders.

Prevention and health promotion strategies that generally are not considered under the purview of clinical psychiatry, such as the promotion of exercise, may have beneficial effects on psychiatric outcomes. For example, some evidence suggests that physical exercise—of clear benefit in the prevention of cardiovascular disease and other chronic medical conditions—may reduce clinical depression and depressive symptoms [19,20].

CHALLENGES FACED BY THE PSYCHIATRIC ADMINISTRATOR APPLYING PREVENTION PRINCIPLES

At least three challenges may present obstacles for administrative psychiatrists interested in promoting prevention. The prevention paradigm is informed meaningfully by the field of public health in addition to medicine, and the relative estrangement between the two disciplines—the former focused on population health and the latter on health care for individuals—is one reason prevention has been relatively underappreciated by psychiatry. In addition to public health, one medical specialty, preventive medicine, focuses on prevention rather than acute treatment and curative medicine. Psychiatric administrators may benefit from collaborations with physicians in the field of preventive medicine, as well as with researchers, educators, and administrators in the public health sector more broadly.

Another difficulty with incorporating prevention that also accounts for the relatively low incorporation of this paradigm is the long-term nature of the outcomes associated with most preventive interventions. Rather than immediate results that seem to justify expenditures of resources and finances fairly acutely, the outcomes of prevention are often quite distant—months, years, or even decades in the future. Indeed, in recent decades, positive results of mental health preventive interventions delivered in childhood have been demonstrated through long-term follow-up using randomized, controlled studies [9]. Similarly, hepatitis B virus vaccination in infancy yields benefits only several decades later. This delay in health returns often makes funding decisions more problematic. Nonetheless, the efficiency and potential cost effectiveness for many well-developed preventive interventions show benefit in terms of ratios of costs to savings. For example, numerous cost-effectiveness analyses have demonstrated the savings and societal benefit associated with widely adopted public health measures, such as routine childhood immunization [21,22].

Still another key challenge associated with applying prevention is that, given the structure of the current health care system in the United States, which is centered on treatment, the issue of who should pay for and who should deliver prevention is debated frequently. Careful consideration of the allocation of limited resources is crucial, given that the public health and medical systems must provide both preventive services and treatment services, although these two sectors are quite separate from one another. It could be argued that there are actually economic disincentives to prevention in the United States. That is, whereas some prosperous countries (eg, the Scandinavian countries) and even some poor countries take a significant percentage of the health care dollar (a finite resource) and in a predetermined fashion direct that portion of fiscal health care resources toward prevention, this allocation is not done in the United States. Thus, administrative psychiatrists face the dilemma of diverting scarce intervention dollars to prevention or not doing prevention at all. These alternatives may create an untenable position for the administrative psychiatrist in charge of and responsible for intervention resources and services. The afore-mentioned optimism of the community mental health movement was related in part to the plan for a portion of funding to be used specifically for prevention services and programs.

The following sections describe some ways in which the prevention para-digm can be incorporated into the varied tasks of administrative psychiatry, despite these challenges. Even if dedicated prevention resources are not avail-able, administrative psychiatrists can still role-model prevention-minded interventions.

THE MEDICAL DIRECTOR'S ROLE IN INCORPORATING THE PREVENTION PARADIGM

Given that administrative psychiatry frequently is the task of the medical direc-tor, the following sections are organized around four tasks commonly performed in this position, whether it be the medical director of a local psychi-atric service (eg, a community mental health center), a county mental health di-rector, a regional or state director of mental health, or a medical director in the private sector (eg, a health maintenance organization). These key roles in which the prevention paradigm can be considered include service delivery, education and training, research, and community consultation and advocacy. Although it can be argued that administration is part of the work of all psychiatrists [23,24], this overview focuses on the ways in which the psychiatrist with a clearly de-fined administrative role can apply the prevention paradigm.

INCORPORATING PREVENTION INTO SERVICE DELIVERY

Administrative psychiatrists typically oversee clinical services and therefore are positioned to encourage the incorporation of prevention principles in the clin-ical setting. Many of the routine practices of clinical psychiatrists are informed partly by the principles of prevention, especially selective and indicated preven-tive interventions [9]. Although administrative psychiatrists generally do not plan or implement population-based prevention and promotion programs, they can encourage providers to practice prevention-minded psychiatry on a daily basis through prevention and promotion interventions for each patient and family seen in the clinical setting [9]. Many clinicians find it very gratifying, and time-efficient, to ask their patients about lead exposure, cigarette smoking, alcohol use, and other matters. Despite obvious divisions between prevention and treatment, administrative psychiatrists can model what is feasible in the clinical setting with individual patients and their families. A number of preven-tion-minded practices can be the focus of service improvement efforts. For example, clinical services can incorporate prevention in one or more of the following areas:

- Early detection of mental illnesses
- Early detection of substance misuse

- Preventing mental illness relapse
- Physical activity/healthy diet/wellness programming
- Preventing substance use comorbidities
- Smoking cessation programs in inpatient and outpatient settings
- Preventing substance abuse relapse
- Suicide prevention

Developments in the field and an overview of the most thoroughly studied prevention and promotion programs have been described in two recent World Health Organization publications, *Prevention of Mental Disorders: Effective Interventions and Policy Options* [2] and *Promoting Mental Health: Concepts, Emerging Evidence, and Practice* [4]. Directors who encourage the inclusion of a prevention perspective in the clinical setting are likely to be seen as progressive and innovative. Just as administrative psychiatry is not divorced from or opposed to clinical psychiatry [23], the prevention paradigm is not separate from or opposed to individual treatment-oriented clinical psychiatry. Many prevention principles can be applied hand-in-hand with general psychiatric practice.

Although service delivery can be influenced at the level of the clinical program, another important way in which service delivery is affected is through policy. Indeed, an important part of administrative psychiatry is policy formulation and decision making [24]. The development of policies affecting a community typically is the function of bureaucratic and legislative authorities, requiring the administrative psychiatrist to move beyond the clinical setting to advance the prevention paradigm further in the domain of service delivery. This responsibility is related to the community consultation and advocacy role of administrative psychiatry discussed later. Administrators can set policy at the program/service level, for example, by encouraging screening for cigarette smoking, substance abuse, depression, and other risks (possibly on electronic patient history templates) or by developing protocols in their institutions for the management of suicidal risk.

THE PREVENTION PARADIGM IN EDUCATION AND TRAINING

Administrative psychiatrists often have an integral role in workforce and leadership development. This role commonly involves responsibilities for the education and training of future psychiatrists and allied mental health professionals. It is vital to include prevention and promotion in curricula for medical students and residents [9]. Just as undergraduate medical education and residency training tend not to provide sufficient training in administration, the prevention paradigm also frequently is neglected in favor of a focus on individual treatment of existing mental illnesses.

Prevention can be incorporated into curricula without minimizing the importance of treating individuals who have mental illnesses. Indeed, the principles of mental illness prevention and mental health promotion should become standard topics of training, as are diagnosis, treatment, and course/outcomes of psychiatric illnesses. Their inclusion will require careful curricular planning, development, and evaluation, given the large and expanding amount of material that already must be covered. In psychiatry residency training, lectures and discussions of specific mental illnesses often begin with statistics on incidence, prevalence, economic impact, and other matters before moving to etiology, phenomenology, diagnosis, and treatment. Including a brief discussion of prevention research and future prospects for preventive interventions will at least engender an attitude of prevention-mindedness. All psychiatric illnesses and substance use disorders should be recognized as potentially preventable conditions—in the future, if not presently—and trainees would benefit from this mindset.

Specialized training in prevention within psychiatry is particularly lacking. Postdoctoral fellowship training is available in a broad array of research areas (eg, mood and anxiety disorders research, psychiatric epidemiology, psychiatric genetics), treatment approaches (eg, cognitive behavioral therapy, electroconvulsive therapy, and psychopharmacology), and overarching paradigms (eg, administrative psychiatry and community psychiatry), in addition to the recognized subspecialties (eg, addictions, child/adolescent psychiatry, consultation/liaison psychiatry, forensics, geriatric psychiatry). Specialized training in prevention for psychiatrists is virtually nonexistent, however. Administrative psychiatrists are in a position to take a lead both in incorporating prevention into existing curricula and in developing new training programs that will promote the prevention paradigm.

BRINGING PREVENTION PRINCIPLES TO PSYCHIATRIC RESEARCH

Psychiatric administrators, who commonly are essential in supporting researchers, can broaden the research portfolio by facilitating prevention-oriented research projects. It could be argued that most psychiatric research informs future prevention goals. Psychiatric administrators, however, may wish to be more progressive by specifically encouraging research that explicitly incorporates prevention-relevant aims and hypotheses. A growing body of research is being produced on preventive interventions, many of which are focused primarily on children, adolescents, and young adults. A large number of preventive interventions have been tested and proven in well-controlled research studies, and focused empiric attention now is being given to the issue of cost effectiveness [3]. In addition to intervention research, studies with obvious preventive implications include more basic clinical research projects, such as those focused on elucidating risk factors and risk markers, as well as protective factors, for psychiatric disorders.

Tertiary prevention-oriented research, beyond treatment trials, also should be promoted, such as interventions to improve treatment adherence in individuals who have serious mental illnesses and programs to promote recovery and reduce disability for those living with a major mental illness. Additionally, broader prevention-focused research that involves people who have mental illnesses also is needed, such as studies on cigarette smoking cessation modalities and interventions to improve dietary composition and physical activity [25]. Developing the evidence base for preventive interventions, whether they are related to primary, secondary, or tertiary prevention goals, requires translating controlled research studies into real-world programs in community sites [9].

Perhaps even more important than promoting prevention-oriented research per se, psychiatric administrators are well positioned to encourage and foster collaboration between psychiatric researchers and prevention researchers. Administrative psychiatrists lead and direct many clinical and educational systems and can influence the people within these systems to value and deepen collaborations that will advance prevention-oriented research.

INCORPORATING PREVENTION-MINDEDNESS IN COMMUNITY CONSULTATION AND ADVOCACY ACTIVITIES

Administrative psychiatrists often work in settings beyond the clinic, and, as suggested previously, promoting prevention often is a task for arenas including advocacy groups, communities at large, legislatures and other bodies that set policies and rules, and professional organizations. Because prevention focuses inherently on populations more than on individuals, prevention is in many cases driven primarily by policy (eg, universal vaccination, standards for prenatal care, rules against advertising cigarettes and alcohol to youth). Just as research must assess carefully the cost effectiveness and economic implications of preventive interventions, policy must address the financing of programs developed to realize preventive, rather than treatment, outcomes. Administrative psychiatrists also can advocate for mental illness prevention and mental health promotion activities when consulting with primary care physicians, health clinics, community agencies, schools, and the workplace, because these are the very settings in which most preventive interventions actually take place [9].

SUMMARY

Prevention psychiatry is a paradigm within psychiatry that focuses on reducing the incidence and prevalence of psychiatric illnesses, substance use disorders, and adverse outcomes related to these conditions (eg, suicide) by identifying risk and protective factors and applying a growing body of evidence-based interventions [9]. As the prevention paradigm develops within psychiatry, designing and evaluating effective prevention efforts and translating results into appropriate, cost-effective changes at the clinical, community, and public/policy levels will be imperative [3]. Because of the high prevalence of mental disorders, the shortage of mental health providers and inadequacy of current services, the great cost of treating these disorders, and the widespread degree of suffering of individuals and their families affected by mental illnesses, it makes sense to work toward preventing disorders and promoting mental health [9]. Leadership is required to address ongoing challenges such as establishing the evidence base of best practices for prevention in psychiatry, clarification of the cost effectiveness of preventive interventions, and determining the most appropriate funding and financing of preventive services.

Acknowledgments

The author expresses his sincere gratitude to the following colleagues who provided advice on this overview: Erica Frank, MD, MPH, Professor and Canada Research Chair, Department of Health Care and Epidemiology and Department of Family Practice, University of British Columbia, Vancouver, British Columbia, Canada; Carol Koplan, MD, Adjunct Assistant Professor, Department of Health Policy and Management and Department of Behavioral Sciences and Health Education, Rollins School of Public Health of Emory University, Atlanta, Georgia; and David Pruitt, MD, Professor and Director of Child and Adolescent Psychiatry, Department of Psychiatry, University of Maryland School of Medicine, Baltimore, Maryland.

References

[1] Mrazek PJ, Haggerty RJ. Reducing risks for mental disorders: frontiers for preventive intervention research. Washington, DC: National Academy Press; 1994.

[2] World Health Organization. Prevention of mental disorders: effective interventions and policy options. Summary report. Available at: http://whqlibdoc.who.int/publications/2004/924159215X.pdf. Accessed October 05, 2007.

[3] Compton MT. Guest editorial: prevention in psychiatry. Psychiatr Ann 2007;37:302–9.

[4] World Health Organization. Promoting mental health: concepts, emerging evidence, practice. Summary report. Available at: http://whqlibdoc.who.int/publications/2004/9241591595.pdf. Accessed October 05, 2007.

[5] U.S. Department of Health and Human Services. Healthy people 2010, chapter 18. Mental Health and Mental Disorders. Available at: http://www.healthypeople.gov/Document/pdf/Volume2/18Mental.pdf. Accessed October 05, 2007.

[6] U.S. Department of Health and Human Services. Agency for Healthcare Research and Quality. Guide to clinical preventive services. Available at: http://www.ahrq.gov/clinic/cps3dix.htm#mental. Accessed October 05, 2007.

[7] President's New Freedom Commission on Mental Health. Available at: http://www.mentalhealthcommission.gov/reports/FinalReport/downloads/FinalReport.pdf. Accessed October 05, 2007.

[8] Substance Abuse and Mental Health Services Administration. National registry of evidence-based programs and practices. Available at: http://nrepp.samhsa.gov. Accessed October 05, 2007.

[9] Koplan C, Charuvastra A, Compton MT, et al. Prevention psychiatry. Psychiatr Ann 2007;37:319–28.

[10] Nurse-Family Partnership. Available at: http://www.nursefamilypartnership.org/index.cfm?fuseaction=home. Accessed October 05, 2007.

[11] Bachrach LL, Clark GH Jr. The first 30 years: a historical overview of community mental health. In: Vaccaro JV, Clark GH Jr, editors. Practicing psychiatry in the community: a manual. Washington, DC: American Psychiatric Press, Inc.; 1996. p. 3–26.

[12] Murray CJL, Lopez AD. The global burden of disease. Cambridge (MA): Harvard University Press; 1996.

[13] Sartorius N, Henderson AS. The neglect of prevention in psychiatry. Aust N Z J Psychiatry 1992;26:550–3.

[14] Compton MT. Considering schizophrenia from a prevention perspective. Am J Prev Med 2004;26:178–85.

[15] Chapman DP, Dube SR, Anda RF. Adverse childhood events as risk factors for negative mental health outcomes. Psychiatr Ann 2007;37:359–64.

[16] Compton MT, McGlashan TH, McGorry PD. Toward prevention approaches for schizophrenia: an overview of prodromal states, the duration of untreated psychosis, and early intervention paradigms. Psychiatr Ann 2007;37:340–8.

[17] Raphael B. Primary prevention: fact or fiction. Aust N Z J Psychiatry 1980;14:163–74.

[18] Durlak JA, Wells AM. Evaluation of indicated preventive intervention (secondary prevention) mental health programs for children and adolescents. Am J Community Psychol 1998;26:775–802.

[19] Larun L, Nordheim LV, Ekeland E, et al. Exercise in prevention and treatment of anxiety and depression among children and young people. Cochrane Database Syst Rev 2006;3:CD004691.

[20] Sjosten N, Kivela SL. The effects of physical exercise on depressive symptoms among the aged: a systematic review. Int J Geriatr Psychiatry 2006;21:410–8.

[21] Deneke MG, Arguedas MR. Hepatitis A and considerations regarding the cost-effectiveness of vaccination programs. Expert Rev Vaccines 2003;2:661–72.

[22] McIntosh ED. Cost-effectiveness studies of pneumococcal conjugate vaccines. Expert Rev Vaccines 2004;3:433–42.

[23] Terhune WB. Administrative psychiatry: a new field—challenging and rewarding. Am J Psychiatry 1957;114:64–7.

[24] Greenblatt M. Administrative psychiatry. New Dir Ment Health Serv 1991;49:5–17.

[25] Compton MT, Daumit GL, Druss BG. Cigarette smoking and overweight/obesity among individuals with serious mental illnesses: a preventive perspective. Harv Rev Psychiatry 2006;14:212–22.

Psychiatr Clin N Am 31 (2008) 85–94

PSYCHIATRIC CLINICS
OF NORTH AMERICA

Telepsychiatry Reduces Geographic Physician Disparity in Rural Settings, But Is It Financially Feasible Because of Reimbursement?

Donald M. Hilty, MD*, Hattie C. Cobb, BA,
Jonathan D. Neufeld, PhD, James A. Bourgeois, OD, MD,
Peter M. Yellowlees, MD, MRCP

Department of Psychiatry and Behavioral Sciences, University of California, Davis,
2230 Stockton Boulevard, Sacramento, CA 95817, USA

G eographic disparities in physician supply have persisted even as the national physician supply has increased steadily, due to economic factors and professional preferences [1]. Programs aimed at recruitment of physicians to rural areas have existed for well over 30 years; most have shown little impact [2]. The federal government, through Title III and Title VII of the Public Health Services Act, has provided scholarships, grants, and loan repayment programs to redistribute health professionals in underserved areas totaling approximately $217 million/year. Rural citizens are still served by roughly half as many physicians per 100,000 as the total United States population, and received only 12% of the decade's physician population increase. In California, physician ratio of non-metropolitan to metropolitan areas is 0.57 (less for generalists at 0.71 and greater for specialists 0.48) [3–5].

Telemedicine facilitates medical care when the patient and health care provider are geographically separated. This separation could be across town, across a region, or even across the world [6]. Telehealthcare in the form of information and communication technologies such as videoconferencing, digital imaging, and electronic data transmission is revolutionizing the practice of medicine [7], and is used for many models of service delivery [8]. Telepsychiatry has clinical efficacy comparable to in-person treatment [9]. Randomized trials show that depression can be successfully treated [10,11]. The number of telemedicine programs declined from 206 in 2001 to 118 in 2004 [12]. This decline is attributed often to a lack of monetary sustainability, which has made it difficult for many telemedicine programs to continue without grant funding, especially in the United States [13].

*Corresponding author. E-mail address: dmhilty@ucdavis.edu (D.M. Hilty).

0193-953X/08/$ – see front matter
doi:10.1016/j.psc.2007.11.010

The cost of telemedicine has been widely debated and discussed, but more recently reimbursement has become important. Bashshur [14] argued that the effects of telemedicine on cost, quality, and accessibility are interconnected, and a comprehensive assessment includes patients, providers, and society. One of the prominent points of contention is how to measure its cost in relation to its effectiveness and/or benefits [13,15,16], but the first systematic meta-analysis of cost found only 38 of 551 articles contained any quantifiable data [17].

Measurements aside, reimbursement for providers remains a challenge, but in California, several rural health networks have arisen to collate and integrate resources and "share" providers, services, and costs. This has improved access to care through telemedicine [18] and accelerated delivery of services, too [19]. The present article reviews the reimbursement rates and payor mix of an e-mental health (e-MH) project, which explored the use of telemedicine for rural service delivery, attempted to get a clear snapshot of whom would be served if all were invited (paying or not), and to understand issues with the reimbursement systems. The study was funded by the California Telemedicine and e-Health Center in Sacramento.

This article (1) examines the receipts of reimbursement and insurance coverage during the 1-year grant period by determining actual versus projected reimbursements, (2) identifies what payor(s) typical patients use, and (3) identifies problems and barriers for future study. Other administrative issues (eg, no-show rates, staffing, scheduling) pertinent to telemedicine and costs are briefly discussed. Clinical outcomes for patients have been previously described [18,19].

METHODS
Participating Partners
Health system
University of California, Davis, (UCD) Health System (UCDHS) is based in Sacramento, California, and encompasses a 33-county area from the geographic center of California to the Oregon state border. UCDHS, through the Center for Health and Technology (CHT), provides telemedical consultations in 28 specialties to 42 clinics (26 rural, 16 prisons) between 100 and 350 miles away. The CHT collaborates with each particular specialty department for services that are needed in these communities.

e-Mental health project
California Telemedicine and e-Health Center funded the UCD Department of Psychiatry and Behavioral Sciences to provide rural mental health services in an e-MH project.

Clinics
Eight rural northern California clinics, defined by the US Census Bureau criteria (http://www.raconline.org/info_guides/ruraldef), would normally require 2 to 6 hours of travel for specialty provider. The sites were the following:

- Colusa Regional Center
- Eastern Plumas Health Care
- Humboldt Open Door
- Hamilton City Clinic
- Madera Family Medical Group
- Oroville Family Health Clinic
- Oroville Hospital
- Plumas District Hospital

All sites had been active users of telemedicine with the CHT previously, except the Oroville Family Health Clinic and the Hamilton City Clinic.

Patients
Of the 298 patients seen in the e-MH project in videoconference, 130 were under age 18 and 52% were female. The majority of the patients seen were white (87%), followed by Hispanic (9%), American Indian (2%), and African American (2%). Of the 165 adult patients, 47% reported being married, 39% single, 9% divorced, 4% widowed, and 2% separated.

Teleconsultation Procedures
Rural primary care providers (PCPs) referred patients to a coordinator on-site for scheduling. Patients were not denied services because of inability to pay, and all ages were accepted. Four psychiatrists and one clinical psychologist at the UCD Medical Center were funded by the e-MH grant. A psychiatric consultation-liaison model was used to provide PCPs with knowledge and help with decision making. Initial and follow-up consultations were 50 and 25 minutes, respectively. Psychotherapy sessions by the psychologist were 50 minutes.

Billing Procedures
All patients seen in the e-MH project (Fiscal Year 2004–2005) for telepsychiatry and telepsychology were abstracted through UCD–CHT according to established UCD billing standards and rates of *Physicians' Current Procedural Terminology, Fourth Edition* established for mental health services. Insurance information was collected at the time of referral, if applicable, and entered into the CHT database. Billing information was submitted to Professional Billing Group (PBG), who billed appropriate payors and recorded and reported all bills and receipts to UCD–CHT.

Services billed included the following:

- Initial psychiatric evaluation, $235
- Psychotherapy (30 min), $117
- Individual psychotherapy (50 min), $158
- Family psychotherapy (without patient present), $155
- Family psychotherapy (with patient present), $184
- Medication management, $84
- Outpatient visit level 2 expanded, $52
- Outpatient visit established level 3 detailed, $73
- Outpatient visit established level 4 moderate, $113

Both public and private insurance reimbursements were examined. Individuals could be covered by a single insurance policy or by multiple policies. Although there is considerable variability among what health insurance companies and state and federal plans cover with regard to mental health services, these are general guidelines that govern much of the reimbursement policies. Public insurance is an insurance plan or policy that is subsidized by federal or state funds (Medicaid, Medicare). To be eligible for these plans, an individual must meet one or more qualifying criteria involving age, income level, and health status. All private insurance is grouped together under the category "third party."

Medi-Cal
The California Medicaid Program provides medical assistance for individuals and families with low incomes and resources. This includes County Medical Services Program and the Medi-Cal Managed Care Program offered by Blue Cross, known as GMC. Rates and conditions are dictated by the California State Plan. Medi-Cal restricts patient co-payments with exception of circumstantial increased income outside of eligibility requirements. Medi-Cal is considered to be "payor of last resort."

Medicare
Medicare is the federal health insurance program for people 65 years of age or older, including certain younger people with disabilities. Medicare coverage is determined by national Medicare policy and is the "payor of first resort."

Medi-Cal–Medicare
Medicare beneficiaries who have low incomes and limited resources may also receive help from the Medicaid Program. For such persons who are eligible for full Medi-Cal coverage, the Medicare health care coverage is supplemented by services that are available under the State's Medicaid Program, according to eligibility category. For persons enrolled in both programs, any services that are covered by Medicare are paid for by the Medicare Program before any payments are made by the Medi-Cal Program, as Medi-Cal is always the "payor of last resort."

Third party
Private insurance is any health insurance policy purchased by an employer or by an individual from a private insurance company. This payor is secondary only to Medicare, as otherwise it is the "payor of first resort." Contractual discounts are negotiated with private insurance providers with health providers based on capitation arrangements.

Data Collection
Three databases (Box 1) were cross-referenced and collapsed for a complete record of all consultations, patients, insurance categories, charges, and receipts.

This project was approved by the Committee on the Protection of Human Subjects at the UCD Medical Center.

Box 1: The three databases used in the e-Mental health project

e-MH database. The e-MH database tracked all patients and consultations, including sociodemographics and services provided in this database in the telemedicine clinic, independently of the CHT.

CHT database. The CHT database tracked all consultations and insurance information of patients seen over telemedicine in an independent database maintained by the CHT through rural site referral forms and clinic coordinator entries of status (completed, no-show, cancellation, reschedule).

INVISION and PBG. INVISION, an appointment tracking program, tracked all appointments of the UCDHS and was automatically extracted by the PBG for billing purposes. In turn, the PBG recorded all bills and receipts. Totals were tallied according to billing code, service provider (psychiatrist versus psychologist), insurance type, collection status (paid, denied, pending), length of pending status (<3 months, 3–6 months, >6 months), and collection rate.

RESULTS

Telemedicine Specific Costs

Technology/equipment

All sites used a videoconferencing system, which consisted of dial-up integrated service digital network lines; transmission speeds of 384 kb/sec; color monitors; Canon pan-tilt-zoom cameras with local and remote control; and a COder-DECoder. The hourly rate for lines ranged from $30 to $60, depending on the distance and long distance carrier. The total capital cost of these videoconferencing units was approximately $6000 to $10,000.

Administrative support

During the e-MH project, the first 6 months were scheduled at UCD (the *provider* site). Estimated administrative time was 50 hours/week; this process included the time of a clinic coordinator, insurance biller, and administrative registration support. The clinic coordinator scheduled patients based on referral arrival with the rural telemedicine coordinator, who in turn scheduled with the patient and provider at a rural clinic. Appointments were often scheduled out 2 months in advance. During the final 6 months, scheduling was done at the *referring* site. The change was necessitated to reduce administrative time at UCD, to provide more control for the rural coordinators in patient scheduling, and to reduce the "no-show rate," which went from 21% to 13%. At the referring site, administrative time was estimated at 20 hours/week. This process included issuing blocked times that are designated to a rural site. The rural site telemedicine coordinator filled the time slot by whatever priority it designated and reported the patient information 2 weeks before appointment date.

Clinical Services

Of the 453 video consultations conducted, 443 (98%) were billed. In addition, 53 consultation bills (12%) have not yet been recorded by PBG owing to recently being billed and a 72-day delay from the consultation date to PBG. Total recorded bills were 390, of which 60% were paid, 30% were pending, 3% were denied, and 8% were uninsured. Of psychiatry (279, 72%) and psychology (111, 28%) consultations, 75% (208) and 32% (36), respectively, were for initial assessment. The average number of consultations per patient was 1.1 for psychiatry and 1.68 for psychology. Psychiatric consultations were mainly for medication management on follow-up. Psychology follow-up visits were mainly for individual psychotherapy (50%) and family psychotherapy (14%).

Reimbursement

Total billed consultations by the primary payor included Medi-Cal (37%), third party (26%), Medicare (24%), and indigent (12%). Cost was split among payors in many cases (Fig. 1), with many patients with a third-party payor themselves

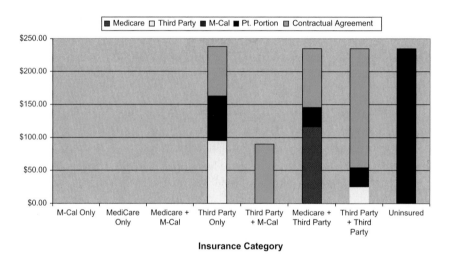

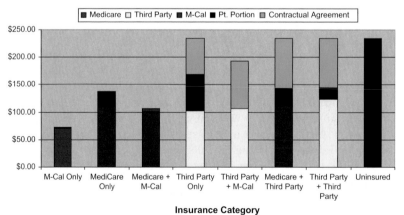

Fig. 1. Initial psychology and psychiatry evaluations per insurance category.

incurring cost. Psychiatrists saw more patients with only Medi-Cal or Medi-care. Average reimbursement by payment type for initial psychiatric and psychological assessment, representing 62% of all consultations, showed a significant disparity in the timeliness of Medi-Cal processing (Fig. 2). Rates of return for total consultations billed under insurance type, represented as paid, currently pending, or denied (Fig. 3), showed the same problem.

DISCUSSION

Not surprisingly, many rural patients are indigent or depend on Medi-Cal or Medicare. This is the first study the present authors are aware of to calibrate whom would likely be served if the "floodgates" were opened and if telemedicine were to be used to attempt to compensate for the rural physician shortage. The trends are concerning—though perhaps not surprising—as rural economies are not strong and the people are underserved in terms of health care and many other dimensions of life. The most serious issue is a high number of indigent, Medi-Cal only, or Medi-Cal/Medicare patients who seemed to be seen by the psychiatrists. This poses a significant financial risk for any party taking on the population without measures to improve the pool of patients or secure contracted rates up front. Though the authors do not know whether the topic has been studied, the concern could get bigger, as in their experience over 11 years, more indigent and Medi-Cal mental health patients are going to the primary care sector on account of a lack of satisfaction with service, stigma, and "more time" with the PCP than the psychiatrist.

Although cost of telemedicine communication charges has decreased, the barrier of reimbursement still stands—no different than any other clinical enterprise—and it disproportionately affects specialties (eg, psychiatry). As many

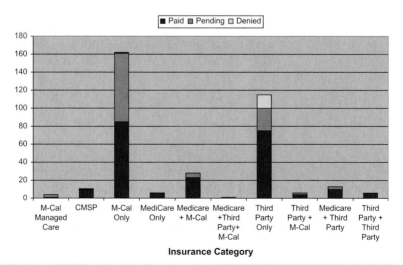

Fig. 2. Status of receipts by payor.

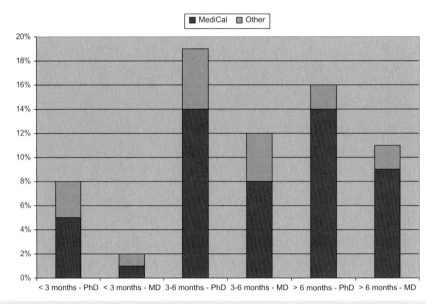

Fig. 3. Percentage of pending bills based on consultant.

administrators know therein, staff attempting to recuperate those funds may spend a disproportionate amount of time on the "tough" payors, those that process more slowly, more detailed requirements, or more denials. The absence of consistent, comprehensive reimbursement policies is often cited as one of the most serious obstacles to total integration of telemedicine into health care practice. Legislation for Medicare over the last 10 years has moved toward expansion of reimbursement policies of telemedicine, including the Balanced Budget Act of 1997 [20] and the Benefits Improvement and Protection Act of 2000 [21]. Currently, 27 state Medicaid programs have full or partial reimbursement for telehealth services, with the most rapid expansion being in the area of behavioral health. Usually, this means reimbursing at the same rate as in-person treatment.

Other streams of reimbursement exist but are not being accessed. County mental health systems are theoretically responsible for mental health care, at least in conjunction with their primary care systems. These systems do not always work well together, and mental health systems often deny telepsychiatry claims, partly to keep costs low and also because the services are provided by someone outside of their system or in the medical sector. This is a problem because patients receive 60% of their mental health services from the medical sector, which they generally prefer owing to less stigma, the ability to maintain an ongoing relationship with their primary care provider, and what is widely perceived to be inadequate care in the mental health sector. Federal programs have been established with high specialist reimbursement for some rural patients, like the Federally Qualified Health Centers and Rural Health Clinics. Telepsychiatry services do not qualify, as consultations are viewed as being provided "outside" the designated clinics.

New models to overcome some financial obstacles are needed, as changing legislation takes significant time. Rural sites working together in health networks helps some, in joining to lobby, access services, and share economic burdens. Resident education may also be an option through academic consultation-liaison (psychosomatic medicine) services, which have been successful in delivering needed care by telepsychiatric providers, as faculty oversee many residents [9]. Consultation-liaison services themselves benefit by expanding the scope of their work to the outpatient sector (eg, contracts for salary and benefits, inpatient reimbursement may be even worse) [22]. Consultation models may have an edge over collaborative care models, which involve more physician time longitudinally [10]. In addition, some health systems with fiscal responsibility over most or all services will employ telepsychiatry, even if reimbursement is poor, as it appears to be cost effective in terms of reducing transfers [23] and hospitalization use [24]. Communities have been able to keep their patients locally, and they have therefore retained dollars that would otherwise have been lost to suburban centers on referral [25].

Limitations of this study include its snapshot of patients over a relatively short period, the fact that rural California may not be representative (eg, 80% white), and that this is not a randomized trial. The study is perhaps more representative of populations, as it surveyed 10 rural sites, including one largely Hispanic.

SUMMARY

Rural populations have a significant number of patients using Medi-Cal and/or who are indigent. Telemedicine is one way to reach these patients, but more research is needed to evaluate methods or models to ensure long-term funding of services because grants eventually run out. In particular, new streams of reimbursement, new collaborations to share financial risk, or new models lowering costs may be needed.

Acknowledgments
The authors thank the University of California, Davis, Department of Psychiatry and Behavioral Sciences, University of California, Davis, Medical Center, Center for Health and Technology, and the California Telemedicine and e-health Center for their support.

References
[1] General Accounting Office Report to theChairman, Committee on Health, Education, Labor, and Pension, US Senate—Physician Workforce. 2003. Available at: www.gao.gov/new. items/d04124.pdf. Accessed December 12, 2007.
[2] Rabinowitz HK, Diamond JJ, Markham FW, et al. A program to increase the number of family physicians in rural and underserved areas: impact after 22 years. JAMA 1999;281(3):255–60.

[3] American Medical Association. Physician Characteristics and Distribution in the US, 2006. Available at: http://www.ama-assn.org. Accessed December 12, 2007.

[4] United States Bureau of Census. Available at: http://www.raconline.org/info_guides/ruraldef. Accessed December 12, 2007.

[5] General Accounting Office. Report to Congressional Requesters. Physician Shortage Areas. Available at: http://www.gao.gov/archive1999/he99036.pdf. Accessed December 12, 2007.

[6] Kennedy C, Yellowlees P. A community-based approach to evaluation of health outcomes and costs for telepsychiatry in a rural population: preliminary results. J Telemed Telecare 2000;6(Suppl 1):S155–7.

[7] May C, Mort M, Mair F, et al. Telemedicine and the future patient: risk, governance and innovation. Innovative Health Technologies. Available at: http://www.york.ac.uk/res/iht/projects/l218252067.htm. Accessed December 12, 2007.

[8] Hilty DM, Yellowlees PM, Cobb HC, et al. Models of telepsychiatric consultation-liaison service to rural primary care. Psychosomatics 2006;47(2):152–7.

[9] Hilty DM, Marks SL, Urness D, et al. Clinical and educational applications of telepsychiatry: a review. Can J Psychiatry 2004;49(1):12–23.

[10] Hilty DM, Marks S, Wegeland J, et al. A randomized controlled trial of disease management modules, including telepsychiatric care, for depression in rural primary care. Psychiatry 2007;4(2):58–65.

[11] Fortney JC, Pyne JM, Edlund MJ, et al. A randomized trial of telemedicine-based collaborative care for depression. J Gen Intern Med 2007;22:1086–93.

[12] Telemedicine Information Exchange. Available at: http://tie.telemed.org/default.asp. Accessed December 12, 2007.

[13] Hilty DM, Bourgeois JA, Nesbitt TS, et al. Cost issues with telepsychiatry in the United States. International Psychiatry 2004;3:6–8.

[14] Bashshur RL. Telemedicine effects: cost, quality, and access. J Med Syst 1995;19(2):81–91.

[15] Grigsby J, Sanders JH. Telemedicine. Where it is and where it's going? Ann Intern Med 1998;129(2):123–7.

[16] Ohinmaa A, Hailey D, Roine R. Elements for assessment of telemedicine applications. Int J Technol Assess Health Care 2001;17:190–202.

[17] Whitten P, Kingsley C, Grigsby J. Results of a meta-analysis of cost-benefit research: is this a question worth asking? J Telemed Telecare 2000;6(Suppl 1):S4–6.

[18] Neufeld JD, Bourgeois JA, Hilty DM, et al. The e-Mental Health Consult Service: providing enhanced primary care mental health services through telemedicine. Psychosomatics 2007;48: 135–41.

[19] Hilty DM, Yellowlees PM, Cobb HC, et al. Use of secure e-mail and telephone psychiatric consultations to accelerate rural health care delivery. Telemed J E Health 2006;12(4):490–5.

[20] Medicare Balanced Budget Act of 1997. Available at: http://www7.nationalacademies.org/ocga/laws/PL105_33.asp. Accessed December 12, 2007.

[21] Benefits Improvement and Protection Act of 2000. Available at: http://www.nmmra.org/providers/review_bipa.php. Accessed December 12, 2007.

[22] Bourgeois JA, Hilty DM, Klein SC, et al. Expansion of the consultation-liaison psychiatry paradigm at a university medical center: integration of diversified clinical and funding models. Gen Hosp Psychiatry 2003;25:262–8.

[23] Alessi N, Rome L, Bennett J, et al. Cost-effectiveness analysis in forensic telepsychiatry: prisoner involuntary treatment evaluations. Telemed J 1999;5(1):17.

[24] Lyketsos C, Roques C, Hovanec L, et al. Telemedicine use and reduction of psychiatric admissions from a long-term care facility. J Geriatr Psychiatry Neurol 2001;14:76–9.

[25] Marcin JP, Nesbitt T, Struve S, et al. Financial benefits of a pediatric care unit based telemedicine program to a rural adult intensive care unit: impact of keeping acutely ill and injured children in their local community. Telemed J E Health 2004;10(Suppl 2):1–5.

Psychiatr Clin N Am 31 (2008) 95–103

PSYCHIATRIC CLINICS
OF NORTH AMERICA

Behavioral Health Electronic Medical Record

Ted Lawlor, MD[a],*, Erik Barrows, MS[b]

[a]Department of Psychiatry, University of Connecticut Health Center, 263 Farmington Avenue Farmington, CT 06030-6410, USA
[b]Enterprise Computing, University of Connecticut Health Center, 263 Farmington Avenue Farmington, CT 06030-5210, USA

The electronic medical record (EMR) is a relatively recent innovation that will (eventually) profoundly impact the practice of all areas of medicine [1]. At present, it is not a universal tool or one embraced by the faint of heart or the traditionalist, but as the younger generation of physicians (who are generally computer and technologically savvy) begin to swell the ranks of practitioners, they will embrace the EMR for its time savings, accuracy, ease of use, and ability to organize information in ways that support multiple service demands and pressures. There are also those time-honored maxims to bear in mind that the first efforts in almost any field of endeavor generally fall far short of the ultimate capabilities of subsequent products, and that the evolution of these offerings can proceed with mind-boggling speed.

Of course, the problem now is that institutional bureaucracies are demanding that EMRs be implemented immediately to meet financial and quality management exigencies [2]. On the face of it, one would not necessarily say that these spurs are any better or worse than any other prompts; however, they have actually led to a narrowing or tunneling of the scope or vision that one hopes for EMRs to attain. This has not only led to initial efforts that are unimaginative and limited in application, but also to fear and loathing amongst some involved physicians as they attempt to conform their practices to new demands or requirements that only partly fulfill their identified needs. A burning question for practitioners is how to break through this glass ceiling and begin having their needs heard, collated, and incorporated into ever-more versatile products.

WHAT DOES THE MODAL PHYSICIAN HOPE FOR?
For those currently faced with using EMRs, there is a broad spectrum of emotions ranging from delight at using a tool that fits with their personal familiarity

*Corresponding author. E-mail address: tlawlor@uchc.edu (T. Lawlor).

0193-953X/08/$ – see front matter
doi:10.1016/j.psc.2007.11.009

and comfort with technological advances, to angst about giving up familiar patterns and habits and entering a realm that may be foreign to them both in the workplace and in their personal life. There are undoubtedly many way stations between these two opposing endpoints. Members of the former group would expect the EMR to enhance their practice by organizing their documentation, laboratory results, investigative procedures, and treatment planning in a concise, readily accessible manner. Those of the latter group would hope that the process would be sufficiently comprehensible and their participation simple enough that they could survive this excursion into the unknown and perhaps even reap some benefit.

WHAT DOES THE DELIVERY OF BEHAVIORAL HEALTH TREATMENT REQUIRE?

The above applies, in some broad, overly inclusive sense, to all areas of medicine, including behavioral health, yet a behavioral health EMR (BH EMR) has to be different from a general medical EMR in particular ways. These include meeting regulatory requirements in a streamlined fashion, doing real quality management, presenting clinical information in a helpful fashion, addressing discipline-specific risk management issues, objectively presenting subjectively gathered data, and facilitating the communication of information across a network of providers.

Meeting Regulatory Requirements in a Streamlined Fashion

One of the issues that bedevils behavioral health practitioners in settings that are licensed and accredited by state and national regulatory agencies, or subject to demands for extra documentation and justification for reimbursement by third-party payers, is the requirements established by these agencies for meeting licensing or accreditation [3]. A BH EMR, appropriately designed and with the requisite logic enabled, can be of great benefit in these instances. In the non-EMR world, the same information must be written a minimum of two times to meet muster—say, in a progress note and a treatment plan. This redundancy serves no purpose other than to meet the requirement that the information be present in at least two different forms as dictated by oversight agencies. No one would argue that it is necessary for the team to think about the issue in question in two separate venues or in two different ways, yet the information must be double documented in whole or in part. The inpatient team meeting is the place where the various practitioners involved in the treatment of an individual patient meet, discuss, and agree on a course of treatment. It does not follow that the outcome of the team's deliberations must be written more than once to make it definitive, cogent, or compelling. That only obtains when the input mode is pen to paper.

In addition, practitioners continue to deal with the issue of how often the treatment plan should be updated or reviewed. General guidelines would suggest that updates occur when a patient is admitted, transferred, or discharged; when a major change occurs in a patient's clinical status; when any treatment goal has been achieved; or when a patient does not achieve treatment goals in spite of good clinical care [4]. On an inpatient service with an average length of stay of less than 1 week, this might well result in frequent updating of the treatment plan. Of course the daily progress note must also reflect the same information. Moreover, when one speaks of documenting the same information "a minimum of two times," it is begging the fact that a discharge form, a medication reconciliation form, an initial or continued stay form for a third-party payer, and the like may also need the same information recapitulated, perhaps along with other repetitive information. The burden on the practitioner begins to defy the expectation that he or she also meets with patients, and all for the same information written repeatedly. An appropriately designed BH EMR eliminates this problem.

Real Quality Management

The title of this section will undoubtedly raise eyebrows, but what is meant by "real" quality management is real-time quality indicators that support the main focus of the clinical enterprise—the care of the patient. Examples of such a program could include parallel processes that query for the input of information or for a change in treatment in response to a guideline- or algorithm-driven approach to patient care management. For the care of an individual patient, this could include reminders that laboratory studies are due; that the present parameters of current treatment modalities are remaining unchanged, although rating scales do not indicate significant improvement in a target condition; and that potential next steps are suggested when a current course of treatment has reached its maximum expected utility, yet response, remission, or recovery is not achieved [5].

On a practice-wide scale, such an approach to quality management would sequester these individual data streams into a data warehouse (particularly if multiple clinical sites are involved) that could be queried at any time to review the outcomes of similar clinical presentations to the myriad (or paucity, or anything in between) of interventions that have been employed. This information could, in its grossest form, display the habits or proclivities of the practitioners involved; show treatment courses generally selected or not selected; display the effectiveness of treatment courses delivered; indicate areas where improvement could be sought; and, in general, support the process that is currently thought of as quality improvement.

There can be a "big brother" feel to being able to oversee any individual caregiver's practice patterns down to such a level of detail; however, in this litigious climate it is a matter of fact that all levels of oversight in a large clinical enterprise are generally deemed responsible and culpable for the actions of the one (or few) practitioner(s) involved in an adverse clinical outcome [6]. However, if oversight of any practitioner's practice patterns is handled judiciously, confidentially (perhaps as part of the peer review process), and with an eye to improving each practitioner's performance in a supportive fashion, it could make an important contribution to bringing evidence-based outcomes to bear directly on the delivery of behavioral health treatment.

Presenting Clinical Information in a Helpful Fashion

The BH EMR should be constructed in a manner that allows for the rapid and accurate assessment of all of the necessary bits of information needed to manage an acute exacerbation or the chronic course of an illness. The logic of the application should be such that information can be sequestered and presented in multiple ways that can be quickly viewed to assist in the care of the patient. An example of this would be multiple disease management programs, constructed by clinicians for clinicians, that include salient signs, symptoms, laboratory values, diagnostic tests, treatment interventions, rating scales, treatment emergent side effects or complications, and concomitant or emergent comorbidities [7]. Having such tools available to manage identified illnesses ensures that the history of course of treatment is immediately available to the caregiver when necessary.

There is a secondary benefit to the presentation of all of the salient details of a course of illness. It is a great teaching tool for the novice clinician and serves as a gentle reminder for the seasoned practitioner. It helps to organize the approach to gathering information and examining the patient [8]. There are those who will argue that such a "cookbook" approach somehow subverts the art of practicing medicine. To those the response would be that physicians are certainly free to interact with their patients in any manner desired; however, the prompts represent minimums that must be met to ensure a consistently appropriate clinical and risk-averse interaction.

Addressing Risk Management Issues

Arguably in general medical and surgical practice, everyone involved (eg, the patient, the practitioner, other clinical disciplines, etc) have all oars pulling in the same direction as they engage in treatment activities. The risk management issues are generally limited to correct diagnosis, appropriate treatment (including informed consent), and, lastly, cost containment of any adverse outcomes [9]. In behavioral health, these same principles solely obtain some fair amount of the time; however, there are also individuals who try to harm themselves or others. These two problems create a whole different world of risk from general medical and surgical practice. To be sure, these two risk areas did not change before and after the advent of the EMR, but using the capabilities of the EMR can mitigate them (and other areas of risk) significantly [10].

This is not to say that these two problems do not occur in settings other than behavioral health; however, the commonly accepted standard of care is that the individual should be kept safe if such a problem is recognized until his or her care is transferred to the behavioral health professional(s). From that point forward, the standard of care that behavioral health professionals are held to is of a much higher order of magnitude. An appropriately constructed BH EMR should have as one of its main components the ability to present historical risk data on any given individual in a manner that supports the real-time evaluation of an individual's risk status. When evaluating risk, the individual's risk history is one of the most important factors to consider [11].

As mentioned in the previous section, the BH EMR should be constructed in such a way as to provide maximum support to the clinical enterprise. From a risk perspective, an added expectation is that the BH EMR should enhance the seamless transition from the primary caregiver to anyone who provides coverage [12]. Although this is an important goal to strive for in all areas of medicine, it is arguably a "must accomplish" in behavioral health as it pertains to risk of harm to self or others. The covering caregiver will likely be held to the standard of complete knowledge of all previously documented risky behaviors and identified risk factors when he or she makes the determination of treatment and level of care [13].

Another area of risk management that the BH EMR should address is the link between patient registration and the tracking of no-shows and cancellations. Although this is undoubtedly handled well in some venues (particularly private practice settings), it is a problem in many outpatient clinic settings. A particular area where it can be most vexing is in training clinics for psychiatry residents that are usually part of a large academic teaching hospital. There are at least two variations to this issue, depending on the EMR that one selects.

In the first instance, the BH EMR is a standalone and must be piped to an already existing patient registration system. This might be attractive from a financial perspective as the existing patient registration application likely serves the hospital as a whole. If this option is selected, desirable reports will probably not be able to be generated by the BH EMR because the bulk of the data necessary to generate them will reside in a data warehouse managed by the patient registration program. This can result in significant obstacles to getting important reports in a timely fashion to help inform responses to no-shows and cancellations.

The second option is to use an EMR with patient registration built into the system. If this were to happen, either one of two kinds of EMR would have to be employed. In the first instance, an institution-wide EMR with patient registration as a subprogram would need to be used. This EMR would have to contain the elements presented in this article to function as a BH EMR. The other choice would be to build an all-inclusive BH EMR that contained a patient registration function, then pipe this to the larger, institution-wide patient registration application. Either of these approaches would allow the patient registration function to be performed within the BH EMR and thus support the generation (in real time) of reports related to arrivals, no-shows, and cancellations.

Objectively Presenting Subjectively Gathered Data

The future of behavioral health care likely includes the collection of self-rating scales during subsequent medication evaluation visits (ie, every medication management visit after the initial intake) as a regular measurement of progress, or lack thereof, in the treatment of identified illnesses [14]. One can debate their value, accuracy, and reliability; however, in contradistinction to the

recollection and documentation of the verbal interview, the patient has committed his or her responses to paper as an enduring record. The other important
benefit is that these rating scales can be completed before the appointment, thus
providing important information immediately to the caregiver in this era of reduced face-to-face time.

The issue then becomes how to convert the subjective information from the
rating scales and the clinical interview into representations that organize it to
make sense of the current clinical encounter as well as compare it with previous
clinical encounters. To be sure, objective data such as laboratory values, diagnostic tests, and findings on physical examination must also be displayed. As
well, a benefit of such an organized display of pertinent information is that
practitioners would be prompted to fill in any gaps they may have created
while collecting data during the course of any particular evaluation.

Facilitating the Communication of Information Across a Network of Providers

This may actually be the most important contribution that a BH EMR can
make to behavioral health care with regard to a large entity such as a state mental health authority (SMHA). The important issue here is that an SMHA assumes responsibility for the behavioral health care of its target or priority
population. Perhaps just as important, each SMHA has the responsibility of ensuring the public safety [15]. What complicates these two responsibilities is that
the provider network that the SMHA employs to carry them out may be com-
posed of a combination of public and private entities [16]. If this is the case, the
mechanisms to share information between providers must be stipulated in the
contractual agreements that exist between the SMHA and the private agencies
for the services they provide [17]. Even if that arrangement is well understood,
honored, and observed, the possibility that important information may be overlooked at a critical juncture unfortunately exists. A BH EMR available at all
times to each agency in the SMHA behavioral health provider network obvi-
ates concerns about the timely communication of all critical information.

The key concept here is that a centralized data warehouse that contains all of
the relevant information about each individual in the target or priority population exists and is continuously updated. In this way, as an eligible individual
moves from site to site within the system for treatment, his or her record
does not just follow, but is immediately available, in its entirety, to the new authorized agency where the individual presents. The benefits of such real-time
access are most apparent during a time of crisis, with potential danger to self
or others being the question evaluated. The instantaneous access to all of the
knowledge in these regards relative to that individual supports the likelihood
of an appropriate clinical (and risk-averse) evaluation and treatment decision.

Of course, appropriate permissions and safeguards must be in place to enable
and preserve the integrity of such a system. The benefits achieved by such complete, instantaneous, and unfettered communication between authorized

caregivers are clearly evident. Both of the SMHA missions of treatment of the individual and ensuring the public safety are enhanced by such a system.

DISCUSSION
Psychiatry, like any other dynamic and fluid field, must constantly review, reevaluate, and reformat itself as new knowledge and greater understanding informs the efforts of psychiatric practitioners. Arguably, this occurs in fits and starts, as some areas of psychiatry show remarkable growth and development (eg, genetics, neuroimaging, psychopharmacology, etc), whereas other practices or tools (eg, the 60-year-old mental status examination, continued reliance on poorly substantiated treatment modalities, employing interventions without fidelity to their precepts, etc) seem to resist change. The latter entrenched entities often have significant cathexis (both positive and negative) attached to them, and they are lightning rods for emotional, rhetorical controversies that defy logic and reason. Attempts to change them are frequently Sisyphean in their denouement.

There are occasional overwhelming external forces, however, that cut through some of the more lugubrious aspects of these unresolved (and seemingly unresolvable) controversies and render the trenchant immediacy of them moot. The most cogent of these usually involves health care financing in some form or other. The last significant example was the ascendancy of managed care as a financing scheme by commercial health insurers. It radically changed the types of addiction services available, greatly impacted the average length of stay of mental health inpatient treatment, and markedly altered the availability of psychotherapy [18,19].

In the case of the EMR, the bureaucratic drive to optimize reimbursement and collect "quality improvement" data is another such prod, this time internally imposed in response to external pressures. Thus, adoption of the EMR is seen as the solution to the need to address fiscal stability and the demands of regulatory agencies for documentation, organization, and consistency in our practice. The EMR is proposed as the (almost) infallible billing mechanism and the apparent end (or the beginning of the end) of the practice of selective, subjective, idiosyncratic documentation of the clinical encounter—another time-honored practice that has so far resisted standardization yet now results in failed regulatory and accreditation visits.

There are significant dangers inherent in such blunt blows to the current practice methods. However, neither of the two listed below should be taken to imply that some type of change is not necessary or desirable. The first is that the solutions proposed often do little more than meet the needs of the bureaucrats who propose them or the agencies that demand them. They do not necessarily enhance how behavioral health treatment is provided or the patients' improvement or satisfaction as a result of it. As well, in their zeal to address their needs, they may force physicians to engage in tasks of little value to themselves but of some benefit to the bureaucracies (eg, checking boxes related to the presence or absence of certain aspects of the mental status examination, relying on boilerplate to incorporate checked boxes into a semblance of narrative, etc). These actions ostensibly meet their needs and enhance professional practice (or so practitioners are led to believe); however, closer examination raises questions as to how limited time and resources could be better spent in the clinical arena.

Another, more important limitation of off-the-shelf, proprietary EMRs is that their sophistication in terms of behavioral health processes is quite limited. It is generally the case that one is given several standard forms (perhaps a progress note and a treatment plan) and encouraged to use a toolbox to modify the EMR to suit one's needs. One has to wonder where the behavioral health experts may have been hiding when these EMRs were constructed. This cursory attention to behavioral health smacks of a parallel process that the commercial insurers used when addressing the behavioral health benefits of their plans—the managed care "carve-outs [20]." Unfortunately, EMRs that have been constructed primarily for use by mental health practitioners are not much more sophisticated.

SUMMARY

The advent of the EMR, although good for all of medicine, will likely reserve its most beneficial effect for behavioral health. It is not likely that the first efforts will be well received—or even deserve to be so. Some examples of them already exist and their frank limitations are apparent. The future is bright, however, particularly if practitioners make all due speed to include the innovations mentioned above. The best news is that these are only some of the advantages that BH EMRs can offer. Contributions to teaching, research, and general improvement in the care that is provided will also become abundantly clear as improvements in the standards of care begin to be seen and the level of skill of practitioners raised. This will not be a smooth, unimpeded progression, but with perseverance and ingenuity much will be accomplished.

References
[1] Institute of Medicine. Crossing the quality chasm: a new health system for the twenty-first century. Washington, DC: National Academies Press; 2001.
[2] Miller RH, West CE. Market watch: the value of electronic health records in community health centers: policy implications. Health Aff 2007;26:206–14.
[3] The Joint Commission website. Comprehensive accreditation manual for hospitals: the official handbook. Standards, rationales, elements of performance, and scoring. 2008.
[4] Kennedy JA. Fundamentals of psychiatric treatment planning. 2nd edition. Washington, DC: American Psychiatric Publishing, Inc.; 2003.
[5] Gilbert DA, Altshuler KZ, Rago WV, et al. Texas medication algorithm project: definitions, rationale, and methods to develop medication algorithms. J Clin Psychiatry 1998;59:345–51.
[6] Beck M. Improving America's health care: authorizing independent prescriptive privileges for advanced practice nurses. University of San Francisco Law Review 1995;29:951–8.
[7] Mays GP, Au M, Claxton G. Market watch: convergence and dissonance: evolution in private sector approaches to disease management and care coordination. Health Aff 2007;26:1683–91.

[8] Osser DN, Patterson RD, Levitt JJ. Guidelines, algorithms, and evidence-based psychophar-macology training for psychiatric residents. Acad Psychiatry 2005;29:180–6.
[9] Reed BJ, Swain JW. Risk management, in public finance administration. Thousand Oaks (CA): SAGE Publications; 1997.
[10] Lawlor T. Suicide Prevention. Presented at Integrating Health Care Systems: Opportunities for Improvements in Suicide Prevention Efforts for Individuals with Serious Mental Illness. National Association of State Mental Health Program Directors. Washington, DC: Medical Directors Council; January 2007.
[11] American Psychiatric Association Practice Guidelines. Practical guideline for the assess-ment and treatment of patients with suicidal behaviors. 2003.
[12] Lawlor T. Public sector risk management: a specific model. Adm Policy Ment Health 2002;29:443–60.
[13] Jablonski v. U.S., 712 F.2D 391 (9th Cir. 1983).
[14] Spitzer RL, Kroenke K, Williams JB. Validation and utility of a self-report version of PRIME-MD: the PHQ primary care study. Primary care evaluation of mental disorders. Patient health questionnaire. JAMA 1999;282:1737–44.
[15] NASMHPD website. Mission and Values Statement. Bylaws, preamble, updated 3/2000. 2008.
[16] Hoge M, Jacobs S, Thakur N, et al. Ten dimensions of public-sector managed care. Psychiatr Serv 1999;50:51–5.
[17] Libby A, Wallace N. Effects of contracting and local markets on costs of public mental health services in California. Psychiatr Serv 1998;49:1067–71.
[18] Goldman W, McCulloch J, Sturm R. Costs and use of mental health services before and after managed care. Health Aff 1998;17:40–52.
[19] Masaquel A, Wells K, Ettner SL. How does the persistence of depression influence the continuity and type of health insurance coverage limits on mental health therapy? J Ment Health Policy Econ 2007;10:133–44.
[20] Salkever DS, Shinogle J, Goldman H. Mental health benefit limits and cost sharing under managed care: a national survey of employers. Psychiatr Serv 1999;50:1631–3.

Psychiatr Clin N Am 31 (2008) 105–122

PSYCHIATRIC CLINICS
OF NORTH AMERICA

Leadership and Professional Workforce Development

Peter F. Buckley, MD[a],*, Vishal Madaan, MD, MBBS[b]

[a]Department of Psychiatry and Health Behavior, Medical College of Georgia, Augusta, GA, USA
[b]Department of Psychiatry and Child Psychiatry, Creighton University/University of Nebraska Medical Center, Omaha, NE, USA

O n an average, 4% of medical students from medical schools in the United States choose psychiatry as an option. Although in recent years psychiatry residency match statistics have improved, in general terms it is less competitive to enter this specialty. Most psychiatrists practice as generalists, either in private practice or in the public mental health system. There are marked shortages in child psychiatry and in upcoming new subspecialties, such as psychosomatics, sleep disorders, and palliative medicine. There are ongoing efforts to enhance the core competency of psychiatrists-in-training, with particular emphasis on research literacy to foster lifelong learning skills and (for some) to stimulate interest in a research career track. This article chronicles the trajectory of workforce development and professional growth in psychiatry.

MEDICAL STUDENTS AND PSYCHIATRY

Medical students constitute the pipeline for and contribute to the vigor of the psychiatry workforce. They are the future leaders in clinical psychiatry and in psychiatric research. It is therefore important to understand factors influencing the recruitment of medical students into psychiatry. Recruitment of medical students into psychiatry in the past has been cyclical and shaped by major developments in psychiatric practice, teaching, and other societal issues [1]. Estimates in the past indicated that only 3.2% of United States medical school graduates chose psychiatry [1]. Similarly, only 5% of Canadian medical graduates ranked psychiatry as their first choice in 2001 [2]. Recent National Resident Matching Program data show that 94.6% of psychiatry positions (1000 out of 1057) were filled, out of which 63.3% were graduates of United States schools [3]. The ratio of available positions to the number of all applicants for whom psychiatry was the first or only choice (0.8) was similar to most other medicine disciplines [3].

*Corresponding author. E-mail address: pbuckley@mail.mcg.edu (P.F. Buckley).

0193-953X/08/$ – see front matter
doi:10.1016/j.psc.2007.11.007

The two aspects of recruitment to psychiatry that have been most studied include (1) an interest in psychiatry, and (2) medical school experiences conducive to choosing psychiatry as a career. Factors that indicate medical student interest in psychiatry include a sensitivity to biopsychosocial aspects of illness, respect for psychiatry, valuing the doctor–patient relationship, understanding the scientific basis of psychiatry, and appreciating the effectiveness of psychiatric treatment [4]. Others have indicated that the best predictor for the number of students matching into psychiatry from a medical school is the proportion of students matching into psychiatry in the prior year for that particular school [5]. In an interesting study comparing the academic performance of psychiatrists compared with other medical specialists before, during, and after medical school, it was found that psychiatrists scored higher on measures of verbal ability and general information before medical school and on evaluations of knowledge and skills in behavioral sciences during medical school, but they scored lower on step 3 of the US Medical Licensure Examination [6].

The issue of increasing medical student recruitment into psychiatry is being addressed at various levels and supported by major academic organizations. The Association of American Medical Colleges (AAMC) has recommended that over the next decade enrollment in accredited medical schools should be increased by 30% from the 2002 level. First-year enrollment in United States medical schools is projected to increase 17% by 2012 to nearly 19,300 students. This expansion should be accomplished by increased enrollment in existing schools and by establishing new medical schools. This increase in medical students should also contribute to the future psychiatric workforce [7].

Similarly, the Psychiatry Student Interest Group Network (www.psychsign. org) was founded in October 2005 by a group of 11 medical students, with direction from Brian Palmer, MD, former president of the American Medical Students Association. With support from the American Psychiatric Association (APA), these students have assembled a network of psychiatry student interest groups with the goal of fostering a community of psychiatric discourse, advocacy, and education among medical students at medical schools across the Untied States and Canada. A similar student interest group is also supported by the American Academy of Child and Adolescent Psychiatry (AACAP) [8].

The APA also organizes a Faculty Development Workshop for Educators' Education. This faculty development workshop is part of the "Educating a New Generation of Physicians in Psychiatry" multiphase project to enhance medical student education in psychiatry [9]. The AACAP also runs a teaching scholars program through the Harvard Macy Institute for Physician Educators Program to fashion master teachers who will inspire medical students and residents to become child and adolescent psychiatrists [10].

Most university programs also have interest groups or neuropsychiatry clubs to elicit medical student interest in the neurosciences generally and to recruit graduates into psychiatry more specifically. Medical students with an interest in psychiatry may benefit from early mentoring at their institutes. There are numerous national mentoring, research, academic, and leadership opportunities available for students to benefit from and enhance and cement their interest in a psychiatry career (Table 1).

There has also been a gradually increasing trend toward stimulating the medical student's interest in psychiatry research. Early experiences in research can not only broaden medical student understanding of the field but also strengthen and integrate early medical education [11]. Various models have been proposed in this regard and range from summer research fellowships and didactics in behavioral health and neurosciences to a structured and mentored clinical neuroscience research training experience. Such structured experiences are mostly institution-specific and may include providing financial support to the medical student to spend a 3- to 12-month block of time in real world clinical research during medical school. Schools with medical scientist training programs (MSTP) must have psychiatrists closely involved with the formal MSTP program. Although details of such models are available elsewhere [11], there is a need for a national initiative to foster and promote medical student interest in basic and translational psychiatry research.

Table 1
Resources for medical students

National Institutes of Health (NIH)
  http://www.training.nih.gov/student/srfp/index.asp
National Institute of Mental Health (NIMH) summer training on aging research
  http://www.psych.org/edu/med_students/startmh.cfm
NIH/Fogarty International Clinical Research Scholars Program
  http://www.aamc.org/students/medstudents/overseasfellowship/
Jeanne Spurlock Minority Medical Student Clinical Fellowship in Child and Adolescent Psychiatry
  http://www.aacap.org/cs/root/medical_students_and_residents/medical_students/awards
Jeanne Spurlock Research Fellowship In Drug Abuse And Addiction for minority medical students
  http://www.aacap.org/cs/root/medical_students_and_residents/medical_students/awards
Program for minority research training in psychiatry
  http://www.psych.org/career_corner/careers_psych/training/summer_oppmed.cfm
Medical student special interest group network
  http://www.psychsign.org/
Child psychiatry special interest group
  http://www.aacap.org/cs/root/developmentor/special_interest_groups
Externship and summer fellowships/travel awards
  http://www.psych.org/career_corner/careers_psych/training/summer_oppmed.cfm
Women health care competencies
  http://wheocomp.apgo.org/
Medical student elective in HIV psychiatry
  http://www.psych.org/aids/medstudent/index.cfm
Association of Directors of Medical Student Education in Psychiatry (ADMSEP) medical student electives
  http://www.admsep.org/studentelectives.html

RESIDENTS IN PSYCHIATRY

Residents in psychiatry constitute the core group that will be future leaders in the field whether as administrators, clinicians, or researchers. The changing demographics of this workforce, the core competencies used for evaluation of training, and recent and proposed changes in the certification process are thus of interest.

Demographics

Recent census data on the characteristics and distribution of psychiatry residents in the United States were released by the APA. Data were collected from the GMETrack, an online survey conducted by the AAMC in collaboration with the American Medical Association. This survey report is based on a 96% response rate from 511 programs accredited by Accreditation Council for Graduate Medical Education (ACGME) for general, child and adolescent, geriatric, forensic, addictions, or combined specialty psychiatry training and psychosomatic medicine. The total number of residents training in psychiatry or one of the subspecialties was 5964, up by 1.08% from the previous year's census [12]. The uneven distribution of the psychiatry workforce continues to be evident, with New York and California leading in numbers of residents while Alaska, Idaho, Montana, and Wyoming had no trainees [12].

Significant findings from this census include an increase in the number of United States medical graduates by 6%, with the number of female residents increasing by 1% from last year to 53%. Combined psychiatry programs showed a higher percentage of men except for the triple board programs in which 63% of residents were female. Whites accounted for the largest percentage of psychiatry residents with the percentage of ethnic minorities staying relatively constant. The number of United States–born residents was almost twice as that residents not born in the United States. The three subspecialties with the highest number of residents were child and adolescent, geriatric, and forensic psychiatry. Psychosomatic medicine, a new subspecialty in psychiatry, had 56% female fellows. Other remarkable findings from the census are listed in Box 1 [12].

Competencies

After the United States Department of Education mandated educational outcome measures for accredited professions, medicine had to define the functions of a physician and associated competencies. This process led to the ACGME identifying six core competencies as dependable means to assess resident performance. The ACGME intention is to ensure that reliable and valid assessment measures be used by training programs to provide "more credible, accurate, reliable and useful educational outcome data" [13]. These competencies represent basic yet essential skills that all residents are expected to learn and display. These core competencies include patient care, professionalism, interpersonal and communication skills, medical knowledge, practice-based learning and improvement, and systems-based practice (Box 2). ACGME has provided a toolbox to assess and evaluate residents (Box 3). There is extensive

Box 1: Salient features of the 2005 psychiatry resident census

Total psychiatry residents: 5964

Gender
Female: 53%
Male: 47%

Race and ethnicity
White: 50.4%
African American: 7.0%
American Indian/Alaska Native: 0.3%
Asian: 24.3%
Native Hawaiian/Other Pacific Islander: 0.5%
Other: 8.3%
Unknown: 9.2%

United States citizenship
United States born: 61.9%
Non–United States born: 34.4%
Unknown: 3.6%

Source of medical training
United States MD: 60.6%
United States DO: 6.8%
International medical graduates (IMGs): 32.6%

Post Graduate Year (PGY) in current program (general psychiatry only)
PGY1: 26.9%
PGY2: 26.0%
PGY3: 26.0%
PGY4: 20.7%
PGY5 and over: 0.4%

Resident enrollment by program type
General psychiatry: 79.5%
Child and adolescent psychiatry: 12.4%
Geriatric psychiatry: 1.7%
Forensic psychiatry: 1.0%
Addiction psychiatry: 0.7%
Psychosomatic: 0.3%
Combined programs: 4.4%

PGY1 positions offered in psychiatry: 1026

PGY1 positions matched in psychiatry: 983
United States seniors matched: 653 (66.43%)
Non–United States seniors matched: 330 (33.57%)

Box 2: Competencies in psychiatry training

ACGME core competencies (ACGME Outcome project):
- Patient care: Compassionate, appropriate, and effective for the treatment of health problems and the promotion of health
- Medical knowledge: Established and evolving biomedical, clinical, and cognate sciences and the application of this knowledge to patient care
- Practice-based learning and improvement: Investigation and evaluation of their own patient care, appraisal and assimilation of scientific evidence, and improvements in patient care
- Interpersonal and communication skills: Effective information exchange and teaming with patients, their families, and other health professionals
- Professionalism: Commitment to performing professional responsibilities, adherence to ethical principles, and sensitivity to a diverse patient population
- Systems-based practice: Actions that demonstrate an awareness of and responsiveness to the larger context and system of health care and the ability to effectively call on system resources to provide care that is of optimal value

Psychotherapy competencies:
- Brief therapy
- Cognitive-behavior therapy
- Combined psychotherapy and pharmacotherapy
- Psychodynamic therapy
- Supportive psychotherapy

information pertaining to the use, psychometric qualities, and feasibility/practicality of each of these tools on the ACGME Web site (http://www.acgme.org/outcome/assess/toolbox.asp) [13,14]. Global ratings are currently the most widely used method of assessment in graduate medical education [13]. Although global rating forms are easy to create and use, they may provide only limited information and direction for remediation.

The challenges for psychiatry residency training programs include expanding on the core ACGME competencies to determine specific and measurable ways to assess psychiatry competencies in general, and psychotherapy competencies in particular. An interesting study by Jarvis and colleagues looked at 13 psychiatric skills to assess how they contributed toward a resident achieving competence. This study concluded that a set of five entries in a resident's portfolio consisting of biopsychosocial formulation, initial evaluation and diagnosis, medical psychiatry, professional communication, and treatment course reflects all competencies with the exception of practice-based learning [15].

Another complex challenge faced by individual psychiatry programs is to develop methods to demonstrate competence of trainees in various forms of psychotherapy, which is important because effective ways to teach psychotherapy

> **Box 3: The Accreditation Council for Graduate Medical Education "toolbox" to assess competence in psychiatry**
>
> - 360-degree evaluation instrument:
> - Chart-stimulated recall oral examination
> - Checklist evaluation of live or recorded performance
> - Global rating of live or recorded performance
> - Objective structured clinical examination
> - Procedure, operative, or case logs
> - Patient surveys
> - Portfolios
> - Record review
> - Simulations and models
> - Standardized oral examination
> - Standardized patient examination
> - Written examination

may not be the best means to assess competence. The American Association of Directors of Psychiatry Residency Training Psychotherapy Task Force developed a list of general psychotherapy competencies that includes basic skills believed to be necessary for all the major forms of psychotherapies (Box 4) [16]. Although implementing such competency assessments is essential, an ongoing evaluation of these measures for their continued suitability is paramount [17].

Although not a part of the core competencies, psychiatry residents across the nation also take the Psychiatry Resident-In-Training Examination (PRITE) every year that provides feedback to the individual residents about the status of their knowledge as compared with others at the same level of training [18]. A recent pilot study trying to establish a relationship between PRITE scores and American Board of Psychiatry and Neurology (ABPN) boards performance found that first-time passers of Boards I and II scored significantly higher on all PRITE global psychiatry categories [19].

Changes and Updates in the Certification Process

The initial certification of residents by the ABPN includes passing a computer-administered examination (Part I) and an oral examination (Part II). Beginning in March 2005, the Part I examination is scheduled for two 3-1/2 hour sessions in the same day and is administered at approximately 200 Pearson VUE testing centers across the United States. Beginning in 2008, the Psychiatry Part I examination will be offered in the spring of the PGY4 year before actual completion of training [20]. This change will impact workforce development especially as more candidates may become board certified earlier than before, which can thus influence the demographics of the post-residency psychiatric practice.

Box 4: General psychotherapy skills (American Association of Directors of Psychiatry Residency Training Psychotherapy Task Force)

Boundaries

Establish and maintain a treatment frame

Establish and maintain a professional relationship

Understand and protect the patient from unnecessary intrusions into privacy and confidentiality

Handle financial arrangements with patients in a manner appropriate to the treatment context

Therapeutic alliance

Establish rapport with a patient

Understand and develop a therapeutic alliance with the patient

Recognize various forms of therapeutic alliances

Enable the patient to actively participate in the treatment

Recognize and attempt to repair disturbances in the alliance

Establish a treatment focus

Provide a holding environment

Listening

Listen nonjudgmentally and with openness

Facilitate the patient talking openly and freely

Emotions

Recognize and specifically describe affect

Tolerate direct expressions of hostility, affection, sexuality, and other powerful emotions

Recognize and describe one's own affective response to the patient

Recognize and tolerate one's uncertainties as a trainee in psychotherapy

Understanding

Empathize with the patient's feeling states

Convey empathic understanding

Resistances/defenses

Identify problems in collaborating with the treatment or the therapist

Recognize defenses in clinical phenomena

Recognize obstacles to change and an understanding of possible ways to address them

Techniques of intervention

Maintain focus in treatment when appropriate

Confront a patient's statement, affect, or behavior

Assess readiness for and manage termination from treatment

Assess patient's readiness for certain interventions

Assess patient's response to interventions

Changes are also being made to the content outline of the part I examination. The applicants for part I should complete training no later than July 31 of that year, must have their program director submit a letter verifying successful completion, and must submit a copy of the full, unrestricted medical license by August 1 [21].

Similarly, part II of the initial certification examination has also undergone various changes, including a switch to numerical scoring in April 2005. More recently, the audiovisual section was replaced by the vignette section (three written vignettes and one video clip) in May 2006. There are plans to replace the patient hour with another vignette in the near future "no earlier than 2008 and no later than 2010 [21]." The rationale for these changes include that patient variability can create difficulties in assessing reliability and fairness of the examination apart from adding expenses to the exam. Furthermore, identification of significant candidate deficiencies in basic competencies after the residency makes remediation difficult [21,22].

In the near future, the ABPN also plans to introduce the need for documentation by the training director of in-residency attainment of specific competencies as a part of the candidate's credentialing process. The specific competencies that need to be evaluated include (1) physician–patient relationship; (2) psychiatric interview, including mental status examination; and (3) case presentation. The ABPN mentions that although resident participation in this evaluation and credentialing process may be voluntary and not required by the ABPN, it may be required by residency programs or the psychiatry residency review committee (RRC). Such a credentialing process would involve the successful completion of three evaluations with any patient type, in any clinical setting, and at any time during residency. Each of these evaluations must be conducted by an ABPN-certified psychiatrist, and at least two of the evaluations must be conducted by different ABPN-certified psychiatrists [21]. ABPN has also signed a contract with BoardPoint to implement a tracking system for resident experiences, including in-residency evaluations [22].

CAREER DEVELOPMENT IN PSYCHIATRY

Demographics

Recent physician specialty data from the AAMC Center for Workforce Studies reveal that psychiatry, with approximately 37,556 active physicians, is fifth among specialties with the largest number of active physicians (Fig. 1) [23]. Psychiatry has a fair representation from the international medical graduates (IMGs) also (Fig. 2). Child and adolescent psychiatry only has approximately 7057 active physicians. Furthermore, these data suggest that the number of people per active physician is around 7900 for psychiatry but 42,300 for child and adolescent psychiatry [23].

Another worrying statistic is that psychiatry has the second highest proportion of active physicians aged 55 or older (approximately 49%) compared with an average of 33.3% across all specialties, again suggesting the need for reinforcing the pipeline of medical students and residents [23]. Psychiatry is fairly

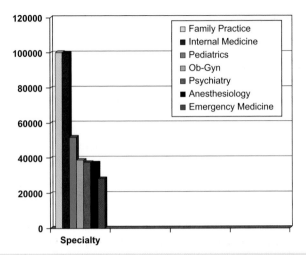

Fig. 1. Specialties with the largest numbers of active physicians. (*Data from* Association of American Medical Colleges. Physician specialty data: a chart book. Center for Workforce Studies, 2006. Available at: https://services.aamc.org/Publications/showfile. cfm?file=version67.pdf&prd_id=160&prv_id=190&pdf_id=67. Accessed September 15, 2007.)

well represented by female active physicians who account for approximately 32% of all psychiatrists and 44% of active child and adolescent psychiatrists compared with an average of 26.7% across all specialties [23].

Other interesting data from the APIRE 2002 National Survey of Psychiatric Practice show that since 1970 psychiatry has grown 86.7%, whereas child psychiatry has grown 194.6%. Psychiatrists are distributed unequally across the country, are working fewer hours than in the past, and less of their time is spent

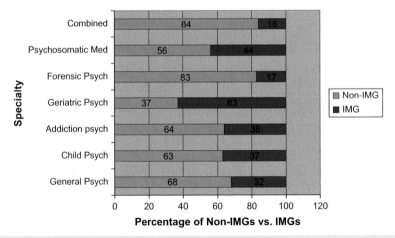

Fig. 2. Percentage of non-IMGs versus IMGs in psychiatry.

in direct patient care activities. It was found that administrative activities claimed an average of 20% of a psychiatrist's time, with a related decrease in time devoted to patient care to 60%. Furthermore, psychiatrists are seeing more patients each week and spending less time with each individual patient. The mean number of patients per week each psychiatrist saw in 2002 was 41 and the mean number of minutes spent with each patient was 34 minutes [24,25].

Although psychiatry is a growing and significant part of the United States physician workforce, trends indicating an aging psychiatric workforce and fewer working hours make it unclear whether psychiatry's current rate of growth will be able to deal with the demand for psychiatric services.

Academic and Research Fellowships

Psychiatry was initially slow to develop subspecialty certification; child and adolescent psychiatry was the only major subspecialty recognized by the ABPN for quite some time. Thereafter, the ABPN recognized additional subspecialties, including geriatric psychiatry, addiction psychiatry, forensic psychiatry, and recently psychosomatic medicine (Box 5). As a primary certifying specialty board, the ABPN has a policy requiring training and certification first in the general field before certification in a subspecialty. The goal has been to keep psychiatry integrated as a practice specialty and academic discipline [20].

The recently conducted APA census (2005–2006) indicates that child and adolescent psychiatry continues to be the biggest subspecialty (Fig. 3; Table 2). Child psychiatry still faces a huge shortage of workforce, however, with the number of people per active physician being 42,300 for child and adolescent psychiatry [23]. Apart from the 2-year fellowship after completing adult training, various training programs also offer integrated programs providing the

---

Box 5: Subspecialty training in psychiatry

Child and adolescent psychiatry: Diagnosis and treatment of developmental, behavioral, emotional, and mental disorders of childhood and adolescence; 2-year program

Addiction psychiatry: Evaluation and treatment of individuals who have alcohol or substance-related disorders, and those who have dual diagnoses of substance-related and comorbid psychiatric disorders; 1-year program

Geriatric psychiatry: Prevention, evaluation, diagnosis, and treatment of mental and emotional disorders in the elderly, and improvement of psychiatric care for healthy and ill elderly patients; 1-year program

Forensic psychiatry: Interrelationships with civil, criminal, and administrative law, evaluation and specialized treatment of individuals involved with the legal system, incarcerated in jails, prisons, and forensic psychiatry hospitals; 1-year program

Psychosomatic medicine: Diagnosis and treatment of psychiatric disorders and symptoms in complex medically ill patients; 1-year program

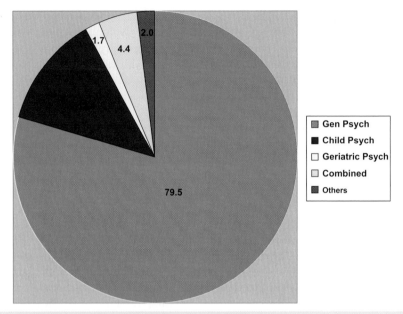

Fig. 3. Resident enrollment by specialty choice, 2005–2006.

resident with early exposure to child psychiatry. Furthermore, approximately 10 programs across the nation provide triple-board residencies for pediatrics-child-adult training also [26].

To address the shortage of child psychiatrists, the AACAP explored the development of a pathway for individuals who have ACGME-accredited training in pediatrics to complete abbreviated training in psychiatry and child and adolescent psychiatry [27]. The RRC for Psychiatry will therefore launch a pilot project to invite up to 10 psychiatry and child and adolescent psychiatry programs to offer a structured 3-year program to train ACGME-trained pediatricians in psychiatry and child and adolescent psychiatry. This project, called the Peds Portal Project, is expected to build on core skills from pediatric

Specialty	APA census	Number of programs
Psychiatry	4742	181
Child and adolescent psychiatry	739	116
Addiction psychiatry	44	42
Forensic psychiatry	58	44
Geriatric psychiatry	104	61
Psychosomatic medicine	16	20
Combined programs	261	46

Table 2
American Psychiatric Association subspecialty census 2005–20006

training without compromising the integrity of traditional resident education in psychiatry and child and adolescent psychiatry, resulting in demonstrated competencies in psychiatry and child and adolescent psychiatry. More information regarding the Peds Portal Project is available on http://www.aadprt.org/news/pppp/Post_Peds_Portal_Project-PPPP.pdf.

The recently started fellowship in psychosomatic medicine is a fully accredited 1-year program for residents entering in their PGY5 year after completion of a general psychiatry residency program [28]. The purpose of this fellowship is to provide competent and comprehensive subspecialty training in consultation-liaison psychiatry. A list of the programs offering this fellowship is available on the Academy of Psychosomatic Medicine Web site at http://www.apm.org/cl-pgms/index.html.

There are numerous other career development opportunities available in the form of clinical research fellowships and clinical scholars programs in neurosciences, schizophrenia, mood disorders, child psychiatry, public psychiatry, HIV psychiatry, and newer methods of treatment, including transcranial magnetic stimulation [29]. More information regarding these opportunities is available at http://www.psych.org/research/apire/res_careerdev/fellowship_opportunities.cfm.

CAREER DEVELOPMENT IN ACADEMICS

The capacity to sustain an academic pipeline in psychiatry is of growing concern. Several years ago, a diverse group called the National Psychiatry Training Council (NPTC) convened in response to an Institute of Medicine report on the difficulty in supporting junior clinical research careers [30]. Although many of the obstacles were thoroughly discussed, the output from NPTC was minimal— perhaps with the exception of endorsing research competency in training (which was then taken up by the RRC). This effort is described earlier in the article. The dilemma of supporting research fellowships and protected research time for junior faculty remains problematic at large, with solutions presently being offered at an individual departmental or institutional level.

It is also noted that the average age of first attainment of a research project grant (RO1) has increased to the mid-40s. Also, the federal research budget has in essence declined over the past 4 years so that institutions have fewer dollars within a more competitive arena. Similarly, although IMGs account for a substantial percentage of the psychiatry physician workforce, they are not eligible to apply for mentored research scientist development grants (K-awards) without having a permanent resident status. A recent innovative program called the Pathway to Independence Awards (K99/R00) may provide these promising postdoctoral scientists an opportunity to receive mentored and independent research support from the same award (http://www.nigms.nih.gov/Training/CareerDev/PathwayIndependence.htm).

These changes are substantial for academic careers, including psychiatry [31]. Some of the more pertinent consequences include a greater emphasis on clinical productivity among faculty, increased emphasis on educator and scholarly (non-research) academic tracks, and a general uncertainly about career expectations (for the individual and the institution). In an effort to provide guidance and support to faculty during this period of academic uncertainty, many medical schools have promoted faculty development initiatives [32] (see www.aamc.org). These range from incentive career funds and support for attending professional development seminars to actual career development centers that provide resources and career counseling to faculty.

An important goal is to retain faculty as productive and engaged members, thereby obviating the demoralization (and considerable expense) of either losing valuable faculty to another institution or their capitulation into private practice. Perusal of psychiatry periodicals reveals plenty of career opportunities in academic psychiatry. Starting on the academic ladder is certainly an accessible option. Succeeding to the top of that ladder is a less certain proposition today [31]. In psychiatry, Roberts and Hilty [33] have produced an excellent text that describes the essentials of career development in academic psychiatry. There are also several key organizations that support professional development (Table 3).

CAREER DEVELOPMENT AND LIFELONG LEARNING

The ABPN, consistent with the overall direction of the American Board of Medical Specialties, has been a forceful proponent for lifelong learning. The board's direction in residency training and initial certification has been described earlier in this article. The ABPN established a time-limited (10 year) certification that requires an examination for recertification and documented evidence of continued medical education (CME) credits. Additionally, it is phasing in a more rigorous Maintenance of Certification (MOC) program that will require evidence of lifelong learning (30 hours of CME per year),

Table 3 Important professional organizations that support career development	
Name	Web site address
Association for Academic Psychiatry	www.academicpsychiatry.org
American Medical Association	www.ama_assn.org
American Psychiatric Association	www.psych.org
American Association of Directors of Psychiatric Residency Training	www.aadprt.org
American Association of Medical Colleges	www.aamc.org
American College of Neuropsychopharmacology	www.acnp.org
American College of Physicians	www.acpoline.org
National Institutes of Health Virtual Career Center	www.training.nih.gov/careers/careercenter

self-assessment activities (one activity beginning in 2010, two activities in 2014), and performance in practice (PIP) (one unit in 2013, two units in 2015, three units in 2017). The following activities are accepted by the ABPN as documentation of lifelong learning:

Psychiatrist in Practice Examination (PIPE)
Post-reading questions from FOCUS
Organized Category 1 CME activities

The PIP evaluation is an independent peer review of practice notes to ascertain whether there is evidence of implantation of knowledge in practice. At the present time, the components of these modules have not been devised. Additionally, the logistics of PIP evaluation are substantial and unclear at present; however, other medical specialties have produced similar programs with success. State licensing boards also require evidence of lifelong learning. Over the years, CME seems to have become a flourishing business. There is great debate as to whether we should continue to have our profession's CME underwritten by the pharmaceutic industry. Missing in this contentious debate is another source of funding for CME.

CME is now obtainable through an ever-increasing array of media. Conferences and symposia remain the backbone of CME. There is now much more emphasis and opportunity for Web-based learning, however. It is likely that this will extend into handheld and other telecommunication media. In fact, numerous new online resources are currently available and easily accessible (Box 6).

There has also been growth in CME-based articles in scientific journals. Keeping an account of all these diverse modalities and the recording/collation of the individual psychiatrist's CME portfolio is challenging. Also, each telecommunication medium for CME has its own strengths and weaknesses and the best admixture of CME (for example, the percentage of web conference versus live CME or web- versus article-based) is presently unclear. This may well become regulated to some extent (just as CME itself is broken down into distinct categories) over time, especially as self-assessment and

Box 6: Online resources for lifelong learning

http://www.pocketpsych.com/Resources/dowloads.htm
http://www.aacap.org/cs/root/member_information/practice_information/
   practice_parameters/practice_parameters
http://www.psychguides.com/
http://www.psychiatryonline.com
http://www.epocrates.com/products/mcme/
http://www.medscape.com
http://www.psychwatch.com/
http://www.e-help.com/psychiatry.htm
http://www.handheldsfordoctors.com

CME-approved activities for MOC programs begin to crystallize. The continued challenge will be to demonstrate how learning has translated into clinical practice.

WORKFORCE NEEDS AND DEVELOPMENT

The mental health needs of America do not match up well with the distribution of our psychiatry workforce. This mismatch is most evident in child psychiatry where there is a large gap between the growing prevalence of psychiatric conditions in childhood and adolescence and the ongoing shortage of child psychiatrists in practice despite recent increased inflow of residents with this subspecialty. Efforts like the Peds Portal Project can help to develop a pipeline into child psychiatry. Increased support for additional graduate medical education training fellowships and support for child psychiatry faculty as educators are needed to achieve workforce expansion here. This area may also be one in which the use of certified psychiatric nurse providers could enhance the provision of service by child psychiatrists. Joint training approaches with pediatrics and family medicine are other alternatives under consideration, wherein the child psychiatrist would function as a tertiary referral–consultation source.

Another obvious area of current shortage in psychiatry is in the Veterans Administration (VA). With estimates that one in five soldiers returning from war have mental health problems, there is a national shortfall in the number of psychiatrists practicing in the VA. The VA has been strategic in providing competitive salaries in its support for program development. It has also allocated funding for mental health fellowship positions. The service expectations have dramatically increased, however, and at academic VA facilities these demands threaten to undermine the academic collaboration between the VA and medical schools that will later yield psychiatrists for the VA. There is presently a Blue Ribbon VA commission addressing this problem (http://www.va.gov/oca/fr/07fe-fr.asp). A detailed description of workforce issues in the VA is available in another article in this issue.

There are other specific gaps in our workforce. For example, career development in administrative psychiatry is ill defined. Most psychiatrists who are in leadership positions reveal that they learned their skills on the job. There are few leadership courses specifically for psychiatrists. There is now an increased emphasis on medical comorbidities in psychiatric conditions. Apart from a handful of medicine–psychiatry training tracks, we are presently ill equipped for this need. It will require a change in curricular emphasis and increasing joint training efforts with medicine and family medicine to address this need. We also have workforce deficiencies that are common to all other specialties. There is insufficient diversity among our psychiatrist workforce. Although matching physician and patient diversity is considered essential in all areas of medicine, it is particularly salient in mental health. The proportion of female clinicians in psychiatry is higher than many other specialties. Women are still underrepresented, however, and this is particularly so among the senior faculty at academic institutions. Other areas of psychiatry are developing career paths that might further expand our field. The American Society of Addiction Medicine is seeking to establish an American Board of Medical Specialties (ABMS) certification in addiction medicine in addition to the already ABPN-approved subspecialty certification in addiction psychiatry. There have also been newly approved certifications in sleep disorders and in palliative medicine, both areas of great psychiatric relevance. On the heels of several national and international disasters, there is now growing interest in disaster psychiatry. Whether this will rise to the level of specialization remains to be seen.

SUMMARY

This article describes the trajectory of career development, beginning with our field's outreach efforts to recruit the most talented into our profession. The article describes regulatory and organized psychiatry initiatives to train and mold the psychiatric workforce to meet the needs of our community. Supply-and-demand discrepancies persist. Addressing these gaps is an important endeavor. Maintaining the academic viability of faculty careers in psychiatry is one key aspect in ensuring the future pipeline of psychiatric clinicians and researchers.

References

[1] Sierles FS, Taylor MA. Decline of U.S. medical student career choice of psychiatry and what to do about it. Am J Psychiatry 1995;152(10):1416–26.

[2] Chandarana P, Pellizzari JR. Canadian perspectives on undergraduate education in psychiatry, in psychiatry in Canada: 50 years (1951–2001). In: Rae-Grant Q, editor. Ottawa (Canada): Canadian Psychiatric Association; 2001. p. 149–61.

[3] NRMP. Results and data. 2007 main residency match. Available at: http://www.nrmp.org/data/index.html. Accessed September 15, 2007.

[4] Manassis K, Katz M, Lofchy J, Wiesenthal S. Choosing a career in psychiatry: influential factors within a medical school program. Acad Psychiatry 2006;30(4):325–9.

[5] Sierles FS, Dinwiddie SH, Patroi D, Atre-Vaidya N, Schrift MJ, Woodard JL. Factors affecting medical student career choice of psychiatry from 1999 to 2001. Acad Psychiatry 2003;27(4):260–8.

[6] Sierles FS, Vergare MJ, Hojat M, Gonnella JS. Academic performance of psychiatrists compared to other specialists before, during, and after medical school. Am J Psychiatry 2004;161(8):1477–82.

[7] AAMC statement on the physician workforce. Available at: http://www.aamc.org/workforce/. Accessed September 15, 2007.

[8] The psychiatry student interest group network. Available at: http://www.psychsign.org/. Accessed September 15, 2007.

[9] Available at: http://www.psych.org/edu/med_students/facultydev.cfm. Accessed September 15, 2007.

[10] Child and adolescent psychiatry teaching scholars program. Available at: http://www.aacap.org/cs/root/research_and_training_awards/child_and_adolescent_psychiatry_teaching_scholars_program. Accessed September 15, 2007.

[11] Balon R, Heninger G, Belitsky R. Medical school research pipeline: medical student research experience in psychiatry. Acad Psychiatry 2006;30(1):16–22.

[12] APA resident census 2005–2006. Available at: www.psych.org/edu/0506census.pdf. Accessed September 15, 2007.

[13] Swick S, Hall S, Beresin E. Assessing the ACGME competencies in psychiatry training programs. Acad Psychiatry 2006;30(4):330–51.

[14] ACGME toolbox. Available at: http://www.acgme.org/outcome/assess/toolbox.asp. Accessed September 15, 2007.

[15] Jarvis RM, O'Sullivan PS, McClain T, Clardy JA. Can one portfolio measure the six ACGME general competencies? Acad Psychiatry 2004;28(3):190–6.

[16] Mellman L, Beresin E, co-chairs AADPRT Psychotherapy Task Force: David Goldberg, Ron Reider, Ron Krasner and Lisa Mellman: Psychotherapy competencies. Further refined by Carol Bernstein and NYU faculty and Hinda Dubin and University of Maryland faculty. Received from aadprt-list@aadprt.org, July 3, 2000.

[17] Bienenfeld D, Klykylo W, Lehrer D. Closing the loop: assessing the effectiveness of psychiatric competency measures. Acad Psychiatry 2003;27(3):131–5.

[18] The Psychiatry Resident-In-Training Examination (PRITE). Available at: http://www.acpsych.org/prite/prite.html. Accessed September 15, 2007.

[19] Roccaforte W, Shostrom V, McArthur-Miller D. Relationships between PRITE and ABPN boards performance. Poster presented at the 36th annual meeting of the American Association of Directors of Psychiatric Residency Training. March 8-11, 2007. San Juan, Puerto Rico.

[20] Initial certification in psychiatry. Available at: http://www.abpn.com/Initial_Psych.htm. Accessed September 15, 2007.

[21] Faulkner LR. The credentialing process for the ABPN. Workshop presented at the 36th annual meeting of the American Association of Directors of Psychiatric Residency Training. San Juan, Puerto Rico, March 8–11, 2007.

[22] Faulkner LR. ABPN certification, recertification, and maintenance of certification: history, current status, and future directions. Newsletter of the American Board of Psychiatry and Neurology, Inc; Spring 2007; 13(1). Available at: http://www.abpn.com/newsletters.htm. Accessed September 15, 2007.

[23] Physician specialty data: a chartbook. Center for workforce studies. Available at: http://www.aamc.org/workforce/. Accessed September 15, 2007.

[24] Scully JH, Wilk JE. Selected characteristics and data of psychiatrists in the United States, 2001–2002. Acad Psychiatry 2003;27(4):247–51.

[25] Mulligan K. Psychiatry workforce trends point to access problems. Psychiatr News 2003;38(14):10.

[26] Available at: http://www.tripleboard.org/. Accessed September 15, 2007.

[27] Available at: http://www.aadprt.org/news/pppp/Post_Peds_Portal_Project-PPPP.pdf. Accessed September 15, 2007.

[28] Available at: http://www.apm.org/cl-pgms/index.html. Accessed September 15, 2007.

[29] Available at: http://www.psych.org/research/apire/res_careerdev/fellowship_opportunities.cfm. Accessed September 15, 2007.

[30] Yager J, Greden J, Abrams M, Riba M. The Institute of Medicine's report on research training in psychiatry residency: strategies for reform—background, results, and follow up. Acad Psychiatry 2004;28(4):267–74.

[31] Heinig SJ, Krakower JY, Dickler HB, Korn D. Sustaining the engine of U.S. biomedical discovery. N Engl J Med 2007;357:1042–7.

[32] Available at: http://www.aamc.org/members/facutlydev. Accessed September 24, 2007.

[33] Weiss RL, Hilty DM. The handbook of career development in academic psychiatry and behavioral sciences. Washington DC: American Psychiatric Press; 2006.

Psychiatr Clin N Am 31 (2008) 123–135

PSYCHIATRIC CLINICS
OF NORTH AMERICA

ELSEVIER
SAUNDERS

The American Board of Psychiatry and Neurology: Historical Overview and Current Perspectives

Stephen C. Scheiber, MD[a], Vishal Madaan, MD, MBBS[b],
Daniel R. Wilson, MD, PhD[b,*]

[a]Department of Psychiatry and Behavioral Sciences, Northwestern University Feinberg
School of Medicine, 446 East Ontario Street, Suite 7-200, Chicago, IL 60611, USA
[b]Department of Psychiatry, Creighton University Medical Center,
3528 Dodge Street, Omaha, NE 68131, USA

The American Board of Psychiatry and Neurology (ABPN) is a nonprofit organization founded in 1934 to serve the public interest and promote excellence in the practice of psychiatry and neurology. This service was to occur principally through its certification and maintenance of certification processes [1]. The ABPN is one of 24 American Board of Medical Specialties (ABMS) boards that have helped develop processes that identify qualified specialists through rigorous credential and training requirements and successful completion of respective certification examinations [2]. The ABPN has had an enormous influence on the practice of psychiatry in America and the world and this influence continues to grow. Here we provide an historical overview of the ABPN, its formation, mission, roles and changes that have taken place over the years in certification, recertification, and maintenance of the certification process.

THE MOVEMENT TOWARD SPECIALIZED MEDICINE
The historical development of the ABPN is linked to the movement for certification and growth of specialty medicine that began in the early 1900s [3]. One of the leading authorities in specialized medicine, Professor Rosemary Stevens, once commented that "specialization is *the* fundamental theme for the organization of medicine in the twentieth century" [4]. This need for medical specialization to assure the community of a specialist's qualifications flourished as successive specialty boards were established. The ABPN, established in 1934, was early in this success and meant to define specialty qualifications and credentials in psychiatry and neurology even as those fields were not yet fully differentiated. The original sponsors included the American Medical Association (AMA), the American Psychiatric Association (APA), and the

*Corresponding author. E-mail address: wilson@creighton.edu (D.R. Wilson).

0193-953X/08/$ – see front matter
doi:10.1016/j.psc.2007.11.008
psych.theclinics.com

American Neurological Association (ANA). These three professional organizations have since continued to serve as nominating societies for the Board, a role in which they were later joined by the American Academy of Neurology and the American College of Psychiatrists (ACP) [1,3].

The ABPN is presently 1 of 24 specialty certifying boards in the United States (Box 1). The American Board for Ophthalmologic Examinations was the first, formed in 1917, followed by the American Board of Otolaryngology in 1924. The Boards in Obstetrics and Gynecology (1930) and thereafter, Dermatology and Syphilology (1932) also preceded formation of ABPN. Another significant development was the foundation in 1933 of the Advisory Board for Medical Specialties that was reorganized in the 1970s as the

---

Box 1: Official American Board of Medical Specialties member boards (year approved in parentheses)

Allergy and Immunology (1971)

Anesthesiology (1941)

Colon and Rectal Surgery (1949)

Dermatology (ABMS Founding Member)

Emergency Medicine (1979)

Family Medicine (1969)

Internal Medicine (1936)

Medical Genetics (1991)

Neurological Surgery (1940)

Nuclear Medicine (1971)

Obstetrics and Gynecology (ABMS Founding Member)

Ophthalmology (ABMS Founding Member)

Orthopaedic Surgery (1935)

Otolaryngology (ABMS Founding Member)

Pathology (1936)

Pediatrics (1935)

Physical Medicine and Rehabilitation (1947)

Plastic Surgery (1941)

Preventive Medicine (1949)

Psychiatry and Neurology (1935)

Radiology (1935)

Surgery (1937)

Thoracic Surgery (1971)

Urology (1935)

Data from the American Board of Medical Specialties. Available at: www.abms.org. Accessed November 16, 2007.

ABMS. The ABMS serves as the umbrella organization that sets standards for member boards and settles jurisdictional disputes [2]. Currently, these 24 ABMS boards certify 37 specialties and 93 subspecialties. Approximately 90% of physicians in the United States are certified by an ABMS-member board, and the rate of certification for United States psychiatrists is at 75% and increasing [2,3].

The ABPN administered its first examination in 1935. The ABPN has since worked to develop processes that identify qualified specialists through rigorous credential and training requirements and successful completion of the Part I (currently computer-administered) and Part II (oral) board examinations for psychiatry, neurology, or neurology with special qualification in child neurology. The ABPN is dedicated to developing tests that assess current scientific knowledge and clinical expertise required to achieve and maintain Board certification [5].

AMERICAN BOARD OF PSYCHIATRY AND NEUROLOGY MISSION AND ROLES

The ABPN was created with the aim to promote excellence in psychiatry and neurology practice through certification and maintenance of certification processes. The board serves the interest of the public and the professions of psychiatry and neurology and describes a physician who has expertise in evaluation, diagnosis, and treatment of patients who have psychiatric and neurologic disorders. The ABPN also sets the standards for knowledge and skills required for certification, administers examinations for evaluations, and monitors and improves the standards and procedures of the certification process. The ABPN also issues certificates and recognizes successful candidates. The ABPN participates in the residency review committee (RRC) of the Accreditation Council for Graduate Medical Education (ACGME) to set standards for the quality and scope of residency training programs and also participates in activities of the ABMS [1].

AMERICAN BOARD OF PSYCHIATRY AND NEUROLOGY STRUCTURE

The ABPN Board of Directors consists of 16 voting members. These members are nominated by professional organizations that include the ACP, APA, AMA, ANA, and the American Academy of Neurology. Although each of these professional organizations proposes nominees to serve on the Board, the Board itself selects its members. Annually, elections are held to replace members whose terms have expired. The Board has an equal representation of neurology and psychiatry despite the considerable numeric preponderance of psychiatrists in practice [1].

AMERICAN BOARD OF PSYCHIATRY AND NEUROLOGY CERTIFICATION: HISTORY AND CURRENT STATUS

ABPN certification is a process designed to assure the larger community that a psychiatrist or neurologist possesses the knowledge, experience, and skills required to provide high-quality patient care. Over the years, requirements for certification have evolved to include an MD/DO degree, completion of an ACGME-accredited residency, attestation by a program director that a candidate has satisfactorily completed training and is able to practice medicine, and successful performance on ABPN examinations.

In keeping with its tradition, the ABPN not only sets the standards for knowledge and skills required for certification in both psychiatry and neurology but also certifies professionals in each specialty. Considering the historical context, most physicians practiced neurology and psychiatry as a combined specialty in the 1930s. Furthermore, the three original sponsors for the board included the APA (clinicians primarily interested in psychiatry and psychoanalysis), the ANA (primarily organic neurologists), and the AMA Section on Nervous and Mental Diseases (clinicians practicing neuropsychiatry). The ABPN continues to certify specialists in both disciplines. The ABPN conducted its first certification examination in 1935 in Philadelphia, administering the examination to 31 candidates. The results from this examination were that 21 examinees passed and 10 failed; 9 candidates were certified in both psychiatry and neurology, 10 in psychiatry only, and 2 in neurology only. The number of specialty certificates awarded since (through 2006) is 44,804 in psychiatry and 12,695 in neurology [1,3,6]. When combined with the number of subspecialty certificates (Table 1), it is clear the ABPN has made outstanding progress from a humble beginning.

The ABPN is the only ABMS Member Board that still uses live patients in the oral (Part II) examinations. In conducting this examination, however, the Board faces many challenges, including assessing reliability resulting from patient variability, extraordinary logistical problems, and great expense. Moreover, remediation for candidate deficiencies after completing residency may be difficult to address. All of these concerns and interests are not always compatible, and the challenge for the ABPN is to attempt to strike a balance among them [7–9].

In an attempt to address some of the concerns, the Board continues to review the initial certification process and initiate major changes. Presently, initial

Table 1
American Board of Psychiatry and Neurology specialty and subspecialty certificates awarded through 2006

Psychiatry	44,804
Neurology	12,695
Child and adolescent psychiatry	6,140
Geriatric psychiatry	2,824
Addiction psychiatry	1,959
Forensic psychiatry	1,594
Psychosomatic medicine	568
Child neurology	1,546

certification of residents by the ABPN includes passing a computer-administered examination (Part I) and an oral examination (Part II). Since March 2005, the Part I examination is administered at Pearson VUE testing centers in different cities across the United States and is scheduled for two 3.5-hour sessions on the same day. Beginning in 2008, the psychiatry Part I examination will be offered in the spring of the Post-Graduate Year-4 (PGY-4) year before actual completion of training. The applicants for Part I should complete training no later than July 31 of that year, must have their program director submit a letter verifying successful completion, and must submit a copy of the full, unrestricted medical license by August 1. Changes are also being made to the content outline of the Part I examination [3,5,7].

Part II of the certification examination has also undergone various changes, including a switch from global to numerical scoring in April 2005. More recently, the audiovisual section (based on a half-hour video of a psychiatric interview) was replaced by four 12-minute case vignette sections (three written and one video clip) in May 2006. Furthermore, there are plans to replace the patient hour with another vignette "no earlier than 2008 and no later than 2010 [7]." The rationale for these changes includes that patient variability creates difficulties in assessing reliability and fairness of the examination apart from adding much to the expense of the exam. The psychiatry certification process will continue to include evaluating clinical skills in the residency, but the psychiatry certification will continue to have a Part I examination followed by a Part II examination using clinical vignettes [1,3,5].

For neurology, assessment of clinical skills will be done during the residency, and successful demonstration of this competency will be one of the credentials for sitting for a 1-day computer-administered examination. This examination will cover the current Part I components and add a clinical vignettes component.

The ABPN regularly notes the results of its examinations in its annual report. Whereas the overall pass rate for Part I was 67% for the years 2001 to 2005, the pass rate for the 1826 candidates in 2006 was 73%. There is a significant difference in the pass rate for new candidates (83%) versus repeat candidates (41%). The overall pass rate of 67% should not unduly concern recent graduates who will be taking the examination for the first time. There is no limit to the number of times a candidate can take the examination. The overall pass rate for the 2006 candidates on the Part II examination was 68%, which contrasted with the 2001 to 2005 pass rate of 55% [1,3]. The pass rate was 62% for new candidates and 45% for repeat candidates. The higher pass rate in 2006 is in part attributable to the new grading system that no longer requires that candidates must pass both sections of the examination. The Board has also instituted a numerical grading system that replaced the pass–condition–fail system of the past. This system is set up as a compensatory one that would allow a candidate who performed brilliantly on one portion of the examination to pass the overall examination, even if marginally failing the other portion. The other significant innovation has been the introduction of four vignettes to replace the audiovisual examination, which allows the candidate to be examined in four different domains in an hour examination. The use of vignettes allows for greater standardization of the examination. Three of these vignettes are written and one is a patient encounter on a video.

The ABPN has cited common reasons for failing the patient section. Examples include a poorly organized history and mental status examination, failure to allow time for a formal mental status examination, premature dismissal of a patient before the allotted 30-minute interview, failure to establish rapport with the patient, and not following up on leads with the patient, particularly regarding suicidality and homicidality.

The ABPN has conducted a study to establish the correlation between passing the Part I and the Part II examinations. The results of this cohort study showed that those who pass Part I on first attempt are somewhat more likely to pass Part II on first attempt [10]. Also those who take the Part I and Part II examinations close to graduation have higher pass rates than those who delay. It is not clear if more able candidates chose to take the examination as soon as possible and less able ones chose to delay sitting for their examinations.

In the near future, the ABPN plans to require documentation by the training director of in-residency attainment of specific competencies as a part of the candidate's credentialing process [11,12]. Specific competencies that will be evaluated include

> Physician–patient relationship
> Psychiatric interview, including mental status examination, and
> Case presentation

The ABPN clarifies that although resident participation in this evaluation and credentialing process may be voluntary (and not required by ABPN), it may be required by residency programs or the psychiatry RRC. This credentialing process would involve successful completion of three evaluations with any patient type, in any clinical setting, and at any time during residency. Each of these evaluations must be conducted by an ABPN-certified psychiatrist, and at least two of the evaluations must be conducted by different ABPN-certified psychiatrists. ABPN has also signed a contract with BoardPoint to implement a tracking system for resident experiences, including in-residency evaluations [5].

RECERTIFICATION AND MAINTENANCE OF CERTIFICATION

Although the ABPN issued a lifetime certificate for successful candidates during its first 60 years of existence, the ABMS mandated a change in the 1990s that allowed the ABPN to issue a 10-year time-limited certificate for General Psychiatry. The ABMS required each of its 24 boards to submit proposals for recertification [2], which necessitated developing measures to recertify diplomates every 10 years, effectively doubling the work of the ABPN. Although there was virtually no rationale for an ongoing contact with lifetime certificate holders, recertification makes it imperative that ABPN establish a lifetime relationship with diplomates who have a time-limited certificate.

In an interesting study on recertification, Choudhry, and colleagues [13] concluded that, "physicians who have been in practice for more years and older physicians possess less factual knowledge, are less likely to adhere to appropriate standards of care, and may also have poorer patient outcomes." The authors explained these results in terms of the ever-changing nature of medical practice and noted that traditional approaches to continuing education have not been effective in changing physician behavior. On the other hand, recertification programs being developed by the members of the ABMS were noted as positive efforts although many of them currently only apply to younger physicians.

With recertification, ABPN expanded its role to include continuing medical education for general psychiatry and each of the subspecialties (Table 2). The ABPN determined it would work with the specialty societies to produce approved educational materials and focus its efforts on certification. A new general psychiatry committee was convened to formulate a content outline and to prepare multiple choice questions for an examination to reflect clinical practice of psychiatry. Similarly, subspecialty committees produced content outlines and prepared examinations to reflect clinical advances in their subspecialties.

Recertification examinations are not meant to replicate initial certification scrutiny. The two differ in that Part I examines basic sciences germane to psychiatry and neurology and topics related to clinical neurology, whereas recertification reflects advances in clinical psychiatry. For this reason, a much higher pass rate on recertification examinations than on the initial certification examinations was anticipated and has held true.

The ABPN, along with other ABMS boards, has expanded recertification processes into maintenance of certification (MOC) (Table 3) [1]. Apart from demonstrating one's professional standing by virtue of licensure and cognitive expertise by testing, the MOC process also involves two new components that include self-assessment and lifelong learning, and assessment of performance in practice. The self-assessment and lifelong learning component is performed in

Table 2
Recertification pass rates (through 2006)

Specialty	No. of examinees	No. passing	Percent passing
Child neurology	80	79	99
Neurology	786	785	99
Psychiatry	1948	1946	99
Subspecialties			
Addiction psychiatry	482	457	95
Child and adolescent psychiatry	300	300	100
Clinical neurophysiology	361	356	99
Forensic psychiatry	272	269	99
Geriatric psychiatry	1162	1100	95

Table 3
Proposed schedule for American Board of Psychiatry and Neurology maintenance of certification requirements

Phase-in schedule for ABPN MOC component requirements (revised 09/29/07)

Original certification year	MOC application year	MOC examination year	CME credits required	First SA activity Required	Second SA activity Required	First PIP unit Required	Second PIP unit Required	Third PIP unit Required
1997	2006	2007	30					
1998	2007	2008	60					
1999	2008	2009	90					
2000	2009	2010	120					
2001	2010	2011	150	X				
2002	2011	2012	180	X				
2003	2012	2013	210	X				
2004	2013	2014	240	X	X	X		
2005	2014	2015	270	X	X	X		
2006	2015	2016	300	X	X	X	X	
2007	2016	2017	300	X	X	X	X	X

Every ABPN diplomate must possess a medical license, and all licenses must be unrestricted. Each SA activity must total a minimum of 100 questions. Only after completing licensure, CME, SA, and PIP requirements are diplomates qualified to complete the ABPN MOC cognitive examination.

Abbreviations: CME, continuing medical education; MOC, maintenance of certification; PIP, performance in practice; SA, self-assessment.

Data from the American Board of Psychiatry and Neurology. Available at: www.abpn.com. Accessed November 16, 2007.

partnership with national psychiatry and subspecialty societies that provide approved educational programs and help track continuing medical education (CME) activities of their members.

After the ABPN had launched its specialties and subspecialties recertification programs, the ABMS introduced a new requirement, MOC. Although recertification included two components (ie, professional standing and cognitive expertise), MOC added two more requirements that included "self-assessment and lifelong learning" and "performance in practice" (PIP) [1]. Although professional standing derives from maintaining an unlimited license to practice medicine, cognitive expertise requires passing an examination that was previously a paper-and-pencil examination but is now a computer-administered examination using a multiple-choice format. These examinations are administered at Pearson VUE testing centers across the nation.

The self assessment and lifelong learning component requires that a diplomate give evidence of participation in at least one self-assessment activity over the 10-year MOC cycle. For completing this requirement, the ABPN has approved the Psychiatrist-in-Practice Examination (PIPE–sponsored by the American College of Psychiatrists), post-reading questions from FOCUS from the APA, the annual self-assessment examination supplement of FOCUS, the APA Practice Guidelines Program, and organized post-CME activities [14,15]. Diplomates are required to complete an average of 30 specialty or subspecialty-specific category I CME credits per year over a 10-year cycle. The implementation of this component is being phased in beginning in 2007.

The fourth component, PIP, will be self-administered. Each diplomate will be required to complete three PIP modules. Each of these modules will require a chart review of five patients who have similar disorders. The diplomate will select a relevant practice guideline from a list of guidelines on the ABPN Web site. After studying the guidelines, diplomates will implement treatment changes in a five-patient sample. To document improvement, diplomates will be required to complete a PIP checklist for each patient. In addition, a PIP summary statement for the entire group must be submitted. If improvement does not occur, a second intervention is required. A second-party external review will also be part of the PIP component.

AMERICAN BOARD OF PSYCHIATRY AND NEUROLOGY SUBSPECIALTY AND COMBINED TRAINING

When founded in 1934, the ABPN took responsibility for certification in general psychiatry and adult neurology only. Yet as we have seen, the board has expanded to include certification in numerous subspecialties, beginning in 1959 with the first child and adolescent psychiatry examination and the first child neurology examination in 1969. In 1988, the ABPN convened interested groups to pursue certification in psychiatric subspecialties. Representatives from six subspecialties–addiction psychiatry, administrative psychiatry, adolescent psychiatry, forensic psychiatry, geriatric psychiatry, and psychoanalysis–met with ABPN psychiatry directors to explore feasibility. An ABPN internal review led to denial of requests to consider administrative psychiatry, adolescent psychiatry, and psychoanalysis as ABPN subspecialties, however. The ABPN also set in motion a request that the field of psychiatry, mostly through the APA, review whether addiction psychiatry, forensic psychiatry, and geriatric psychiatry were appropriate as new subspecialties.

ABPN approval for geriatric psychiatry was accelerated when ABMS approved a new subspecialty in geriatric medicine for diplomates of the American Board of Internal Medicine and the American Board of Family Practice (now Family Medicine). This acceleration was because of a concern that psychiatrists would not get Medicare funding for the subspecialty and thus would not be on a par with internists and family medicine geriatricians. ABPN thus initiated and sped up efforts to approve geriatric psychiatry, with the first subspecialty examination taking place in 1991 [16].

In the past 15 years, ABPN has played a key role in shepherding approval of new subspecialties directly with ABMS and indirectly with ACGME. ABPN has greatly expanded the number of subspecialties to include clinical neurophysiology, addiction psychiatry, forensic psychiatry, psychosomatic medicine, neurodevelopmental disabilities, vascular neurology, psychosomatic medicine, and pain medicine (with the American Boards of Anesthesiology and Physical Medicine and Rehabilitation) (Table 4) [17–22].

Most recently, ABMS has approved certification in sleep medicine (with the American Boards of Internal Medicine, Pediatrics, and Otolaryngology) and neuromuscular medicine (with the American Board of Physical Medicine and Rehabilitation). The ABPN has joined with the American Boards of Internal Medicine, Family Medicine, Pediatrics, Physical Medicine and Rehabilitation, Surgery, and Anesthesiology in applying to the ABMS to issue a subspecialty certificate in Hospice and Palliative Medicine.

Table 4
American Board of Psychiatry and Neurology subspecialty approval

ABMS approval	First examination	Subspecialty
a	1959	Child and adolescent psychiatry
1989	1991	Geriatric psychiatry
1990	1992	Clinical neurophysiology
1991	1993	Addiction psychiatry
1992	1994	Forensic psychiatry
1998	2000	Pain medicine
1999	2001	Neurodevelopmental disabilities
2003	2005	Psychosomatic medicine
2003	2005	Vascular neurology
2005	Scheduled 2008	Neuromuscular medicine
2005	Scheduled 2007	Sleep medicine
2006	Scheduled 2008	Hospice and palliative medicine

aCertificates issued before 1972 when ABMS recognition procedures were established.
Data from the American Board of Psychiatry and Neurology. Available at: www.abpn.com. Accessed November 16, 2007.

In addition to subspecialties, the APBN negotiated with other boards for combined training in two or more specialties. These programs allow graduates to sit for each of the board certification examinations usually with abbreviated training in each of the specialties. In particular, the board has a longstanding tradition of recognizing combined training programs in psychiatry and neurology.

In 1986, the ABPN joined forces with the American Board of Pediatrics (ABP) and the National Institute of Mental Health to sponsor an experimental program of combined integrated training in pediatrics, psychiatry, and child and adolescent psychiatry. This "triple board program" was set up to bridge the gap between specialties and to enhance the care of children who have mental illness. Six programs were accepted for study and were intensively evaluated over a 10-year period. This program included 2 years of pediatrics, 18 months of general psychiatry, and 18 months of child and adolescent psychiatry. After 10 years, this unique program was given permanent status by the ABPN and the ABP [23,24]. Similarly, a pilot Post-Pediatrics Portal Project has just begun for pediatricians interested in certification for General and Child–Adolescent Psychiatry [25].

Other combined training programs include Psychiatry and Internal Medicine, Psychiatry and Family Medicine, Neurology and Internal Medicine, Neurology and Physical Medicine and Rehabilitation, and Neurology–Diagnostic Radiology–Neuroradiology. Typically, the total training is reduced by 1 year in these combined programs. The board discontinued combined training in Neurology and Nuclear Medicine when no individuals chose to enter that combined training program [26–28].

AMERICAN BOARD OF PSYCHIATRY AND NEUROLOGY: OTHER INITIATIVES

The ABPN has also taken a leadership role in numerous other initiatives and academic pursuits. The board has been involved in recording and updating core competencies in psychiatry and neurology. In June 2001, the board convened a meeting with leaders in Canadian and American psychiatry and neurology to establish core competencies for both disciplines, which resulted in the publication of two seminal works, one for each discipline. As a result, all test questions for ABPN examinations in both disciplines and in all subspecialties are now linked to core competencies.

The ABPN also serves as one of the three appointing bodies to the RRC for psychiatry. Usually, three general psychiatrists and two child and adolescent psychiatrists from each of the three appointing bodies including the ABPN, the APA, and the AMA serve on the RRC. The ABPN is also strongly represented at the American Association of Directors of Psychiatric Residency Training (AADPRT) annual meetings. The ABPN directors, staff, and the executive vice president lead workshops, take part in plenary sessions, and update the attendees with the latest changes being brought on by the board.

The ABPN also invested in a major research and development effort in the late 1990s, namely experimenting with the use of standardized patients for its examinations. Although the ABPN has not used standardized patients for testing purposes, there is still a possibility that they will be used to develop vignettes for the Part II examination.

The ABPN also was a pioneer in building its own computer test center in Deerfield, Illinois, which allowed the ABPN to administer its small cognitive examinations on computer and to host the other two boards (along with other boards interested in administering the computer-based tests). This led to the ABPN's subsequent contract with Pearson VUE to administer all of its cognitive examinations at computer test centers. This contractual relationship with Pearson VUE allows 90% of candidates to sit for computer-administered examinations within 100 miles of where they live and practice.

Another significant political success for the ABPN was the arrangement negotiated with the Royal College of Physicians and Surgeons of Canada to allow diplomates who are licensed in one of the provinces of Canada to seek ABPN certification. Likewise, American diplomates with a license in one of the states or territories can apply for Canadian certification. This reciprocity agreement was based on certification, not on training.

SUMMARY

The ABPN is one of the ABMS boards that serves the public interest and promotes excellence in the practice of psychiatry and neurology through its certification and maintenance of certification processes. The ABPN has played a major role in graduate education in psychiatry and neurology since 1934. Established as a consequence of the process of specialization of medicine, the ABPN has currently established itself not only as the certifying body in psychiatry, neurology, and their subspecialties but also as a connecting force between the professional organizations, such as the APA, AACAP, AADPRT, ACGME, ABMS, the training programs, the trainees, and clinicians needing recertification. The ABPN continues to progress toward and fine tune its certification and recertification processes. With maintenance of certification it faces the challenge to achieve the same level of relevance with CME and lifetime learning. The future success of the ABPN will depend on its ability to continue to nurture its professionals in psychiatry and neurology as it moves toward implementing future changes in its certification processes.

References
[1] ABPN. Available at: www.abpn.com. Accessed November 16, 2007.
[2] ABMS. Available at: www.abms.org. Accessed November 16, 2007.
[3] Scheiber SC. ABPN: past, present and future—its impact on American psychiatry. Omaha (NE): Grand Rounds, Creighton University Medical Center; 2007.
[4] Stevens R. American medicine and the public interest. Berkeley (CA): University of California press; 1998. p. 1–600.
[5] Faulkner LR. ABPN certification, recertification, and maintenance of certification: history, current status, and future directions. Newsletter of the American Board of Psychiatry and

Neurology, Inc.; 2007;13(1): Available at: http://www.abpn.com/newsletters.htm. Accessed November 16, 2007.

[6] Juul D, Scheiber SC, Kramer TA. Subspecialty certification by the American Board of Psychiatry and Neurology. Acad Psychiatry 2004;28(1):12–7.

[7] Faulkner LR. The credentialing process for the ABPN. Workshop presented at the 36th Annual Meeting of the American Association of Directors of Psychiatric Residency Training. San Juan (PR), March 8–11, 2007.

[8] Quick SK, Robinowitz CB. Examination success and opinions on American Board of Psychiatry and Neurology certification. Am J Psychiatry 1981;138(3):340–4.

[9] Moran M. New ABPN executive sees big changes for board exam. Psychiatr News 2006;41(10):10.

[10] Juul D, Scully JH Jr, Scheiber SC. Achieving board certification in psychiatry: a cohort study. Am J Psychiatry 2003;160(3):563–5.

[11] Scheiber SC, Kramer TA, Adamowski SE. The implications of core competencies for psychiatric education and practice in the US. Can J Psychiatry 2003;48(4):215–21.

[12] Scheiber SC, Juul D, Adamowski S. The ABPN core competencies: what they are, where they came from, how they are being used. ACGME Bulletin, Feb 2004. p. 5–7.

[13] Choudhry NK, Fletcher RH, Soumeria SB. Systematic review: the relationship between clinical experience and quality of health care. Ann Intern Med 2005;142:260–73.

[14] FOCUS. Available at: http://focus.psychiatryonline.org/index.dtl. Accessed November 15, 2007.

[15] American Psychiatric Association. Available at: www.psych.org. Accessed November 15, 2007.

[16] Juul D, Scheiber SC. Subspecialty certification in geriatric psychiatry. Am J Geriatr Psychiatry 2003;11(3):351–5.

[17] Aminoff MJ, Massey JM, Scheiber SC, et al. Certification in neuromuscular medicine: a new neurologic subspecialty. Neurology 2007;68(14):1153–4.

[18] Adams HP Jr, Biller J, Juul D, et al. Certification in vascular neurology: a new subspecialty in the United States. Stroke 2005;36(10):2293–5.

[19] Palmer FB, Percy AK, Tivnan P, et al. Certification in neurodevelopmental disabilities: the development of a new subspecialty and results of the initial examinations. Ment Retard Dev Disabil Res Rev 2003;9(2):128–31.

[20] Juul D, Percy AK, Kenton EJ 3rd, et al. Board certification in child neurology and neurology: cohort study. J Child Neurol 2005;20(1):25–7.

[21] Percy AK, Juul D, Scheiber SC, et al. Certification in child neurology: new directions for the twenty-first century. J Child Neurol 2005;20(8):644–7.

[22] Bloom JD, Benson JA Jr. Subspecialization in psychiatry: third-generation programs. J Am Acad Psychiatry Law 2005;33(1):95–8.

[23] Schowalter JE, Friedman CP, Scheiber SC, et al. An experiment in graduate medical education: combined residency training in pediatrics, psychiatry, and child and adolescent psychiatry. Acad Psychiatry 2002;26(4):237–44.

[24] Changes in ABPN recertification and maintenance of certification in child and adolescent psychiatry. American Board of Psychiatry and Neurology [special communication]. J Am Acad Child Adolesc Psychiatry 2002;41(1):106–8.

[25] AADPRT News. Post Peds Portal project. Available at: http://www.aadprt.org/news/pppp/default.aspx. Accessed December 7, 2007.

[26] Doebbeling CC, Pitkin AK, Malis R, et al. Combined internal medicine-psychiatry and family medicine-psychiatry training programs, 1999–2000: program directors' perspectives. Acad Med 2001;76(12):1247–52.

[27] Carney CP, Pitkin AK, Malis R, et al. Combined internal medicine/psychiatry and family practice/psychiatry training programs 1999-2000: residents' perspectives. Acad Psychiatry 2002;26(2):110–6.

[28] Rachal J, Lacy TJ, Warner CH, et al. Characteristics of combined family practice-psychiatry residency programs. Acad Psychiatry 2005;29(5):419–25.

Psychiatr Clin N Am 31 (2008) 137–147

PSYCHIATRIC CLINICS
OF NORTH AMERICA

Psychiatry: Organized and Disorganized

Stuart Munro, MD[a], Daniel R. Wilson, MD, PhD[b],*

[a]Department of Psychiatry, University of Missouri-Kansas City School of Medicine, 1000 East 24th Street, Kansas City, MO 64108, USA
[b]Department of Psychiatry, Creighton University Medical Center, 3528 Dodge Street, Omaha, NE 68131, USA

> Professional Societies form a living matrix where minds meet and engage and where trusted colleagues pool their knowledge, helping each other to glimpse and plumb larger forces at work, to see connections among events, and to imagine the future.
>
> Janet Bickel [1]

Human beings have a natural tendency to relate to one another through the formation of social groups. Originally, perhaps, the bond was familial for the purpose of preservation of the clan. Later, cohesive forces became more complex and diverse. Thus it is not surprising the common property of being a psychiatrist and working in a particular area of the field serves as one such cohesive force.

Psychiatry is relatively young as a formal area within the field of medicine. Although there is a long tradition of medical approaches to disturbances of behavior and emotion (Hippocrates' humoral theory is one example), physicians who concentrated their life's work on such challenges were rare and often were on the margins of medical practice. The Victorian term for such eccentrics—"Alienist"—surely implicated the practitioner along with the patient. Physicians who focused their work on the mentally ill also found themselves competing with the shaman, the faith healer, and the like. In this unpromising context, forming an organization was one way to establish and preserve professional identity.

One such physician in early America was Benjamin Rush, who frequently has been described as "the father of American psychiatry." Rush recommended a wide variety of mechanical and chemical interventions for disturbances of behavior and emotion that have failed the test of scientific analysis. Nonetheless, he was a prolific inventor and writer within the emerging field of mental health treatment. The largest grouping of American psychiatrists (perhaps the

*Corresponding author. E-mail addresses: wilson@creighton.edu; wilson-322@cox.net (D.R. Wilson).

0193-953X/08/$ – see front matter
doi:10.1016/j.psc.2007.11.003

largest such group in the world), the American Psychiatric Association, takes his profile as their logo.

Table 1 is a timeline of the origins of some of the prominent organizations within the field.

The American Psychiatric Association (APA) was founded in 1844 [2]. It may well be the oldest psychiatric organization in the United States, and it certainly can claim the largest current membership, more than 35,000, as well as the greatest impact on psychiatry throughout the globe. Attendance at recent annual scientific meetings is in the tens of thousands, with as many as a third of the participants traveling from other countries. The organization suffers from its size and the generic nature of its membership, however. In a recent communiqué to members (M.T. Lymberis; APA Elections Survey; e-mail communication to all members of the American Psychiatric Association on August 10, 2007), the APA Elections Committee recognized the problem of declining membership participation in the electoral process. The e-mail message reported the number of members voting in the national election has been eroding steadily from its height of 59% in 1968 to the present low of 28% in 2007. The APA also sponsors an annual Institute for Psychiatric Services that typically is another of the best-attended psychiatric meetings in America. The APA manages what probably is the largest psychiatric publishing house in the world. While serving as the largest national psychiatric organization, the APA impacts communities at the local level through district branches and state associations and at the regional level through seven Area Councils. In its District Branch/State Association Directory [2] the APA lists at least one such organization for each state. The only states with multiple listings are New York, which has 13, California with six, Missouri, oddly, with three, and New Jersey with two. Clearly these numbers are influenced as much by historical accident as by population density. The District of Columbia also has an affiliated psychiatric society, as do Puerto Rico and the Uniformed Services. Three Canadian psychiatric societies are also affiliates. "Psychiatric Society" and "District Branch" are common names for these organizations; alternatives used by some states include "Psychiatric Medical Association" and "Psychiatric Physicians Association."

The remaining national psychiatric organizations can be grouped together by several common purposes or themes.

EDUCATION
The American Association of Chairs of Departments of Psychiatry (AACDP) is one of the oldest psychiatric organizations focused on academic psychiatry [3]. Until the mid-1960s, the organization was essentially an eating club [4]. John Romano (University of Rochester) became the organization's first president in 1963. Mickey Stunkard (University of Pennsylvania) drafted the first constitution in 1965. The first dues were established in 1967 at $25 per year. Of the 38 presidents, 9 also have served as president of the APA. Four schools have been represented more than once. When Laura Roberts became the

President-elect in 2006, she was the first woman elected by the organization, even though 6 of the last 23 APA presidents have been women.

Several years ago, the AACDP identified the need for a manual or "tool kit" designed to help a new chair get started. The group soon realized that a close relative, the American Association of Directors of Psychiatric Residency Training (AADPRT), had outpaced the AACDP. In 2003, AADPRT members, along with the Executive Administrator, Lucille Meinsler, produced an excellent orientation manual for new members in their organization [5]. This document served as a good model as the AACDP Tool Kit [6] was developed. Similarities in format and component parts are discernable to the keen observer.

The AADPRT is one of the most vibrant and influential of psychiatric organizations related to education. When Iago Gladstone became the first president in 1970, membership was limited to directors of residency programs, but since then the organization has relaxed its membership criteria and broadened its constituency [7]. At the 2007 annual meeting in Puerto Rico, 271 program directors and associate program directors participated along with 52 residents and 88 residency program coordinators (personal communication, Lucille Meinsler, AADPRT, 2007). Similarly, the Association of Directors of Medical Student Education in Psychiatry (ADMSEP), founded in 1975 [8], was initiated by a membership defined by its role within academic departments of psychiatry. Although associate directors, coordinators, residents, and students are welcome to attend the annual meeting, these gatherings typically have been more intimate than those of AADPRT. The Association for the Behavioral Sciences and Medical Education also focuses on the education of medical students and residents [9] but has a broader membership, including medical school faculty in a variety of disciplines.

The Association for Academic Psychiatry (AAP), founded in 1974 [10], attracts membership more generally from academia, although many participants in the annual meeting are deeply engaged in the education of residents and medical students [11]. These four organizations that follow the education theme (AACDP, AADPRT, ADMSEP, and AAP) together sponsor a journal titled *Academic Psychiatry*. The March/April 2007 issue featured a series of articles about a variety of psychiatric organizations [12] and serves as a fine companion to this review of psychiatric organizations.

The American College of Psychiatrists (the "College") is an honorary association of psychiatrists who have been recognized for their significant contributions to the profession [13]. Membership is limited to 750 practicing psychiatrists who have achieved national recognition in clinical practice, research, academic leadership, teaching, or leadership in psychiatry. New members must be nominated by current members. Members are expected to attend at least one of every three annual meetings. The College has a major impact on residency training through the Psychiatric Resident-in-Training Examination that it conducts annually for all residents in psychiatry nationwide. This examination provides residents and their training program directors with a reliable gauge of their preparedness to sit for the written component of the specialty board examinations [14]. Similarly, the College produces a Child Psychiatric

Table 1
Partial timeline of organization founding with acronyms and Websites

Year	Organization	Acronym	Website
1841	Royal College of Psychiatrists	RCP	rcpsych.ac.uk
1844	American Psychiatric Association	APA	psych.org
1911	American Psychoanalytic Association	APsaA	apsa.org
1924	American Orthopsychiatric Association	AOA	01,968bc.netsolhost.com
1929	Royal College of Physicians and Surgeons of Canada	RCPSC	rcpsc.medical.org
1934	American Board of Psychiatry and Neurology	ABPN	abpn.org
1942	American Group Psychotherapy Association	AGPA	groupsinc.org
	American Psychosomatic Society	APS	psychosomatic.org
1945	Society of Biological Psychiatry	SOBP	sobp.org
1946	Group for the Advancement of Psychiatry	GAP	groupadpsych.org
1950	World Psychiatric Association	WPA	wpanet.org
1951	Canadian Psychiatric Association	CPA	cpa-apc.org
1953	American Academy of Child and Adolescent Psychiatry	AACAP	aacap.org
	Academy of Psychosomatic Medicine	APM	apm.org
1956	American Academy of Psychoanalysis and Dynamic Psychotherapy	AAPDP	aapsa.org
1959	National Association of State Mental Health Program Directors	NASMHPD	nasmhpd.org
1961	American College of Neuropsychopharmacology	ACNP	acnp.org
1963	American Association of Chairs of Departments of Psychiatry	AACDP	aacdp.org
	American College of Psychiatrists	The College	acpsych.org
1967	American Society for Adolescent Psychiatry	ASAP	adolpsych.org
1969	Association for the Behavioral Sciences and Medical Education	ABSAME	absame.org
	Black Psychiatrists of America	BPA	blackwebportal.com
	American Academy of Psychiatry and the Law	AAPL	aapl.org
1970	American Association of Directors of Psychiatry Residency Training	AADPRT	aadprt.org
1974	Association for Academic Psychiatry	AAP	academicpsychiatry.org
1975	Association of Directors of Medical Student Education in Psychiatry	ADMSEP	admsep.org
	American Academy of Clinical Psychiatrists	AACP	aacp.com

(continued on next page)

Year	Organization	Acronym	Website
Table 1 *(continued)*			
1978	American Association for Geriatric Psychiatry	AAGP	aagpgpa.org
1983	National Foundation for Depressive Illness (became the American Society of Clinical Psychopharmacology [ASCP] in 1992)	NAFDI ASCP	ascpp.org
	Association of Women Psychiatrists	AWP	womenpsych.org
1984	American Association of Community Psychiatrists	AACP	comm.psych.pitt.edu
1985	American Academy of Addiction Psychiatry	AAAP	aaap.org
	Association of Gay and Lesbian Psychiatrists	AGLP	aglp.org
1987	NASMHPD Research Institute	NRI	nri-inc.org
1988	American Neuropsychiatric Association	ANPA	anpaonline.org
1990	American Association of Organizational and Occupational Psychiatry	AOOP	aoop.org
1991	Association of Medicine and Psychiatry	AMP	amedpsych.com
1995	Psychiatric Society for Informatics (became the American Society for Technology in Psychiatry in 2002)	AATP	techpsych.org
1998	Academy of Cognitive Therapy	ACT	academyofct.org

Adapted from Mueller T, McCarthy M, Levy BR, et al. Membership orientation manual. Hartford (CT): American Association of Directors of Psychiatric Residency Training; 2003. p. 48–56.

Resident-in-Training Examination and provides a Web-based Psychiatrists In-Practice Examination that practicing psychiatrists find useful in their lifelong learning endeavors as well as for maintenance of certification through the American Board of Psychiatry and Neurology (ABPN).

The Group for the Advancement of Psychiatry was founded in 1946 by a group of physicians, led by William Menninger, whose wartime experiences convinced them of the need for greater public awareness of the need to improve the approach to mental health issues in the United States [15]. Membership is by invitation only. Three hundred psychiatrists are divided into 29 committees that select their own topics for exploration, analyze data, invite participation by expert consultants from other disciplines, and present the resulting work to the entire membership of the Group for the Advancement of Psychiatry for further scrutiny. Frequently, the results include published reports, videotape presentations at scientific meetings, and other means of dissemination.

CLINICAL SPECIALTY

Areas of specialization within the field of psychiatry run the gamut of patient age, diagnosis, and point of service setting. In terms of age, childhood attracted specialization within the field earlier than did the special needs of older populations. For example, the American Academy of Child and Adolescent Psychiatry was founded in 1953 [16], and the American Society for Adolescent Psychiatry was founded in 1967 [17]. By contrast, the American Association for Geriatric Psychiatry was not founded until 1978 [18]. Likewise, the first added qualifications examination in child psychiatry was offered by the ABPN in 1959, whereas a similar offering in geriatric psychiatry did not occur until 1991 [19].

There are numerous excellent national advocacy groups whose mission includes seeking to improve the lives of persons suffering from a variety of mental illnesses. In that they do not exclusively or predominantly seek psychiatrists for membership, they do not fall under the scope of this review. A number of organizations for psychiatrists focus on specific areas of diagnostic interest, however, including the American Academy of Addiction Psychiatry [20], the American Academy of Psychiatry and the Law [21], the Academy of Psychosomatic Medicine [22], the American Psychosomatic Society [23], and the Association of Medicine and Psychiatry [24]. The last three also could be considered to focus on practice setting, in this case on the interface between psychiatry and other specialties within the field of medicine. Other organizations themed by point of service setting include the Academy of Organizational and Occupational Psychiatry [25], the American Academy of Clinical Psychiatrists [26], the American Association for Emergency Psychiatry [27], and the American Association of Community Psychiatrists (AACP) [28].

When the National Association of State Mental Health Program Directors (NASMHPD; pronounced "nash-pid") was founded in 1959 (personal communication, Joe Parks, NASMHPD, 2007), most state mental health commissioners were psychiatrists who acted as a combined agency CEO and medical director [29]. The increasing complexity of health care systems and the accompanying demands on their administrators required increased sophistication with political, administrative, and fiscal skill sets that were well beyond the administratively inclined psychiatrists, who lacked formal management experience and training. Apart from some elements of anti-psychiatry ideology, states responded by recruiting non-psychiatrist commissioners with formal management training and experience. Today, NASMHPD represents the $26 billion public mental health service delivery system, serving more than 6 million people annually in all 50 states, four territories, and the District of Columbia. The NASMHPD Research Institute (NRI) was established in 1987 [30] with the stated mission of promoting the quality and accountability of mental health services by generating and facilitating the use of relevant research, data, and information that meets the collective and individual needs of state mental health authorities. In fact, many mental health care organizations outside the purview of state mental health authorities rely heavily on the NRI database.

RESEARCH

Organizations have formed within the field of psychiatry to provide a forum for presentation and critique of emergent research work as well as a catalyst for ideas regarding new areas of discovery. Included in this category is the American College of Neuropsychopharmacology [31], which maintains archives of its publications that can be accessed via the Vanderbilt University Website [32]. Another such organization is the American Society of Clinical Psychopharmacology (ASCP), which has produced a model curriculum of psychopharmacology for residents in psychiatry that now is in its fourth edition [33]. The ASCP originated as the National Foundation for Depressive Illness. Further examples in this category include the American Neuropsychiatric Association [34] and the Society of Biological Psychiatry [35] that publishes the journal *Biological Psychiatry*, ranked sixteenth among 200 neuroscience titles on the 2005 Institute for Scientific Information Journal Citations Reports. The American Association for Technology in Psychiatry, formerly known as the Psychiatric Society for Informatics, represents one of the newer waves of discovery within the field [36].

THE PSYCHIATRIST'S IDENTITY

Most countries of the world are represented by physicians who have immigrated to the United States to train and practice in the field of psychiatry. There is a formal or informal communication network and gathering of these psychiatrists by each country of origin. Psychiatrists who are international graduates applauded the election of George Tarjan to the Presidency of the APA in 1983. He was the first international graduate to serve in that capacity in the modern era [2]. The Department of Minority/National Affairs within the APA administers a number of Minority/Underrepresented Group Caucuses. The APA Website currently lists the American Indian/Alaska Native/Native Hawaiian Caucus; the Asian-American Caucus; the Black Caucus; the Hispanic Caucus; the Lesbian, Gay, and Bisexual Caucus; the International Medical Graduates Caucus; and the Women's Caucus. Apart from the APA, a number of organizations reflect the personal characteristics of the members. These include the Association of Gay and Lesbian Psychiatrists [37], the Association of Women Psychiatrists [38], and Black Psychiatrists of America [39], to name a few.

TREATMENT MODALITY

Perhaps influenced by historical divisions within the field regarding approaches to treatment, numerous organizations represent specific treatment modalities. Examples include the Academy of Cognitive Therapy [40], the American Academy of Psychoanalysis and Dynamic Psychiatry [41], the American Group Psychotherapy Association [42], the American Orthopsychiatric Association that endorses a multidisciplinary approach to treatment [43], and the American Psychoanalytic Association [44]. Organizations focus on biologic approaches to treatment have been reviewed in the Research section. Also of note is the APA Caucus on Complementary, Alternative and Integrative Care initiated in 2004 [2].

CERTIFYING ORGANIZATIONS AT HOME AND ABROAD

Any review of psychiatric organizations should include the ABPN, the body that certifies qualified specialists in the fields of psychiatry and neurology [19]. The current association of the two specialties is a reflection of an historical intertwining of the fields. Sigmund Freud trained as a neurologist at the Salpetriere Institute in France. Charcot was his teacher, and Babinski was a fellow student. The ABPN was founded in 1934, following conferences of committees appointed by the APA, the American Neurological Association, and the then Section on Nervous and Mental Diseases of the American Medical Association. Although the written examination component of the certification process in psychiatry retains a significant sampling of purely neurologic questions, the practical examination component, by design, no longer involves the evaluation of a patient with a specifically neurologic condition. In fact, the duration of the ordeal of live patient evaluation has been significantly, and mercifully, shortened in the decades since the certification process was initiated. The emergence of examinations for added qualifications in the subspecialties of child and adolescent psychiatry (1959), geriatric psychiatry (1991), addiction psychiatry (1993), forensic psychiatry (1994), psychosomatic medicine (2005), and sleep medicine (scheduled for 2007) reflects the evolution of the field, and more subspecialties are on the way. In recruiting examiners for candidates' demonstration of clinical competence, the ABPN has included a broad spectrum (age, gender, geographic location, practice setting) of practitioners in the field.

The Royal College of Psychiatrists offers an interesting cross-Atlantic comparison [45]. Established in 1841, 3 years before the APA, the Royal College serves as the main professional organization of psychiatrists in the United Kingdom and the Republic of Ireland. Like the ABPN, the Royal College is responsible for certifying psychiatrists (the pathway to the MRCPsych degree). The organization also addresses psychiatric training at all levels and public policy and disseminates information regarding mental health issues. It publishes many books and several professional journals, including the *British Journal of Psychiatry*. The organization originally was known as the Association of Medical Officers of Asylums and Hospitals for the Insane; the name subsequently was changed to the Medico Psychological Association. The Royal Charter was bestowed in 1926.

Specialty certification of Canadian psychiatrists is managed by the Royal College of Physicians and Surgeons of Canada [46], an organization that also assumes responsibility for accreditation of residency programs in all specialty areas. The Canadian Psychiatric Association (CPA), founded in 1951, is self-described as the national voluntary professional association for Canada's 4000 psychiatrists [47]. The CPA's mission is to forge a strong, collective voice for Canadian psychiatrists and to promote an environment that fosters excellence in the provision of clinical care, education, and research. There are other Royal College cognate entities around the world, including Australia and New Zealand.

The World Psychiatric Association (WPA) traces its roots to 1950 when the first World Congress of Psychiatry was held in Paris [48]. The organization was known at the time as the International Society for the Organization of World Congresses of Psychiatry. The president, Jean Delay, and Secretary General, Henry Ey, were French. It was 1957 before the second World Congress was held in Zurich. Since then, 11 World Congresses have been convened. Only one has been held in the United States (in Hawaii in 1977). The formal founding of the WPA occurred in 1961. The first American president, Howard Rome, was elected in 1972. He had served as President of the APA from 1965 to 1966. Juan Mezzich of the United States was elected Secretary General of the WPA in 1996 and currently serves as President. A permanent headquarters, or Secretariat, has been established near Geneva.

ANALYSIS

Do psychiatrists affiliate with each other more effectively than do their colleagues in other specialties? Should they be expected to do so because of their training in a field that focuses on emotions and behavior and the dynamic qualities of human relationships? The first question must remain rhetorical until comparative studies are undertaken, and the second may provide good fodder for debate. The collaboration between the AACDP, AADPRT, AAP, ADMSEP, and APA to produce the journal *Academic Psychiatry* is a good example of the benefits of groups working together for a cause. An international example is the collaboration between American psychiatrists, under the auspices of the APA, and psychiatrists from around the globe working with the World Health Organization on integrating the *Diagnostic and Statistical Manual* with the International Classification for Diseases. For this project, field trials were conducted at 151 clinical centers in 32 countries by 942 clinician/researchers who conducted 11,491 individual assessments of patients [49].

At the annual scientific meeting of the APA held in Toronto, Canada in May, 2006, an event of note occurred [50]. Then APA President Steven Sharfstein and WPA President Juan Mezzich chaired a symposium titled "International Advocacy Toward Psychiatry for the Person." This gathering embodied a spirit of international cooperation sorely needed outside the field of psychiatry. A speaker from Malaysia discussed person- and community-centered organization of services in developing countries, a speaker from Peru discussed advocacy for women's and children's mental health, and a speaker from Norway reviewed international advocacy for patients' human rights. There were other speakers from Great Britain, Greece, and beyond.

With all their opportunities for affiliation, psychiatrists should be among the professional groups most effective in administration, at least as the word derives from the Latin compound of *ad* ("to") and *ministratio* ("give service"). Certainly through the decades, both for good and for ill, psychiatrists have tried to organize people and their resources efficiently to achieve common goals. As the means of and venues for professional affiliation in psychiatry grow ever more elaborate, perhaps the profession and its increasingly diverse constituents will progress toward ever better consequences in patient care, teaching, and research.

References

[1] Bickel J. The role of professional societies in career development in academic medicine. Acad Psychiatry 2007;31:91–4.

[2] American Psychiatric Association. Available at: http://www.psych.org/about_apa/. Accessed September 10, 2007.

[3] American Association of Chairs of Departments of Psychiatry. Available at: http://www.aacdp.org/web/public/contact.html. Accessed September 5, 2007.

[4] Munro S. A tool kit for new chairs. Acad Psychiatry 2006;30:301–3.

[5] Mueller T, McCarthy M, Levy BR, et al. Membership orientation manual. Hartford: American Association of Directors of Psychiatric Residency Training; 2003.

[6] Munro S, Meinsler L. Tool kit for new chairs. Hartford: American Association of Chairs of Departments of Psychiatry; 2004.

[7] American Association of Directors of Psychiatry Residency Training. Available at: http://www.aadprt.org/aadprt/exec_office.aspx. Accessed September 5, 2007.

[8] Association of Directors of Medical Student Education in Psychiatry. Available at: http://www.admsep.org/history.html. Accessed September 5, 2007.

[9] Association for the Behavioral Sciences and Medical Education. Available at: http://www.absame.org/info/absinfo.htm. Accessed September 5, 2007.

[10] Association for Academic Psychiatry. Available at: http://www.hsc.wvu.edu/aap/. Accessed September 5, 2007.

[11] Worley L. The unique role of psychiatric organizations and societies in professional development. Acad Psychiatry 2007;31:112–3.

[12] Weerasekera P. Psychiatric organizations: influencing professional development. Acad Psychiatry 2007;31:89–90.

[13] American College of Psychiatry. Available at: http://www.acpsych.org/prite/prite.html. Accessed September 10, 2007.

[14] Webb LC, Juul D, Reynolds CF, et al. How well does the Psychiatry Residency In-Training Examination predict performance on the American Board of Psychiatry and Neurology Part I Examination? Am J Psychiatry 1996;153:831–2.

[15] Group for the Advancement of Psychiatry. Available at: http://www.groupadpsych.org/files/aboutgap. Accessed September 5, 2007.

[16] American Academy of Child and Adolescent Psychiatry. Available at: http://www.aacap.org/cs/root/about_us/about_us. Accessed September 5, 2007.

[17] American Society for Adolescent Psychiatry. Available at: http://www.adolpsych.org/. Accessed September 5, 2007.

[18] American Association for Geriatric Psychiatry. Available at: http://www.aagponline.org/about/downloads/AAGP25th_anniv1.pdf. Accessed September 5, 2007.

[19] American Board of Psychiatry and Neurology. Available at: http://www.abpn.com/mission.htm. Accessed September 5, 2007.

[20] American Academy of Addiction Psychiatry. Available at: http://www.aaap.org/about-us.htm. Accessed September 5, 2007.

[21] American Academy of Psychiatry and the Law. Available at: https://www.aapl.org/org.htm. Accessed September 5, 2007.

[22] Academy of Psychosomatic Medicine. Available at: http://www.apm.org/about/mission-vision.shtml. Accessed September 11, 2007.

[23] American Psychosomatic Society. Available at: http://www.psychosomatic.org/. Accessed September 5, 2007.

[24] Association of Medicine and Psychiatry. Available at: http://www.amedpsych.com/modules/news/. Accessed September 5, 2007.

[25] Academy of Organizational and Occupational Psychiatry. Available at: http://www.aoop.org/aboutus.shtml#02. Accessed September 5, 2007.

[26] American Academy of Clinical Psychiatrists. Available at: http://www.aacp.com/. Accessed September 5, 2007.

[27] American Association of Emergency Psychiatrists. Available at: https://www.emergencypsychiatry.org/. Accessed September 5, 2007.

[28] American Association of Community Psychiatrists. Available at: http://www.comm.psych.pitt.edu/mission.html. Accessed September 5, 2007.

[29] National Association of State Mental Health Program Directors. Available at: http://www.nasmhpd.org/about_us.cfm. Accessed September 5, 2007.

[30] NASMHPD Research Institute. Available at: http://www.nri-inc.org/aboutus/index.cfm. Accessed September 5, 2007.

[31] American College of Neuropsychopharmacology. Available at: http://www.acnp.org/. Accessed September 5, 2007.

[32] Nature Publishing Group. Available at: http://www.nature.com/npp/index.html. Accessed September 5, 2007.

[33] American Society for Clinical Psychopharmacology. Available at: http://www.ascpp.org/?q=node/65. Accessed September 5, 2007.

[34] American Neuropsychiatric Association. Available at: http://www.anpaonline.org/. Accessed September 5, 2007.

[35] Society of Biological Psychiatry. Available at: http://www.sobp.org/purpose.asp. Accessed September 5, 2007.

[36] American Association of Technology in Psychiatry. Available at: http://www.techpsych.org/about.htm. Accessed September 5, 2007.

[37] Association of Gay and Lesbian Psychiatrists. Available at: http://www.aglp.org/pages/chistory.html. Accessed September 5, 2007.

[38] Association for Women in Psychiatry. Available at: http://www.womenpsych.org/member.html. Accessed September 5, 2007.

[39] Black Psychiatrists of America. Available at: http://www.blackwebportal.com/yellow/dt.cfm?ID=531. Accessed September 5, 2007.

[40] Academy of Cognitive Therapy. Available at: http://www.academyofct.org/FolderID/1054/SessionID/%7BC56B07C7-D63F-48E1-B9C6-70CA3EBE7DDE%7D/PageVars/Library/InfoManage/Guide.htm. Accessed September 5, 2007.

[41] American Academy of Psychoanalysis and Dynamic Psychotherapy. Available at: http://aapsa.org/academy_membership.html. Accessed September 5, 2007.

[42] American Group Psychotherapy Association. Available at: http://www.agpa.org/. Accessed September 5, 2007.

[43] American Orthopsychiatric Association. Available at: http://01968bc.netsolhost.com/PastandPresent.htm. Accessed September 5, 2007.

[44] American Psychoanalytic Association. Available at: http://apsa.org/ABOUTAPSAA/tabid/55/Default.aspx. Accessed September 5, 2007.

[45] Royal College of Psychiatrists. Available at: http://www.rcpsych.ac.uk/college/whatwedo.aspx. Accessed September 5, 2007.

[46] Royal College of Physicians and Surgeons of Canada. Available at: http://rcpsc.medical.org/tools/sitemap_e.php. Accessed September 5, 2007.

[47] Canadian Psychiatric Association. Available at: http://ww1.cpa-apc.org:8080/About/About_CPA.asp. Accessed September 5, 2007.

[48] World Psychiatric Association. Available at: whttp://www.wpanet.org/home.html. Accessed September 5, 2007.

[49] Sartorius N, Ustun TB, Korten A, et al. Progress toward achieving a common language in psychiatry, II: Results from the international field trials of the ICD-10 diagnostic criteria for research for mental and behavioral disorders. Am J Psychiatry 1995;152:1427–37.

[50] Sharfstein SS, Mezzich JE, Cox JL, et al. APA-WPA Presidential Symposium on International Advocacy Towards Psychiatry for the Person. Available at: http://www.psych.org/edu/other_res/lib_archives/archives/meetings/AMS/2006saps.pdf. In: Programs and abstracts of the 159th Annual Scientific Meeting of the American Psychiatric Association. Toronto: 2006. Accessed September 18, 2007.

Psychiatr Clin N Am 31 (2008) 149–155

ELSEVIER
SAUNDERS

PSYCHIATRIC CLINICS
OF NORTH AMERICA

INDEX

0193-953X/08/$ – see front matter
doi:10.1016/S0193-953X(08)00009-9